Clinical Effectiveness in Practice

edited by

Carol Lynn Cox and Adrian Reyes-Hughes

palgrave

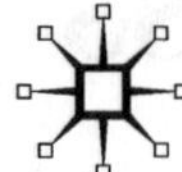

First published 2001 by
PALGRAVE
Houndmills, Basingstoke, Hampshire RG21 6XS and
175 Fifth Avenue, New York, N. Y. 10010
Companies and representatives throughout the world

PALGRAVE is the new global academic imprint of St. Martin's Press LLC Scholarly and Reference Division and Palgrave Publishers Ltd (formerly Macmillan Press Ltd).

ISBN 0–333–80455–4 paperback

This book is printed on paper suitable for recycling and made from fully managed and sustained forest sources.

A catalogue record for this book is available from the British Library.

10 9 8 7 6 5 4 3 2 1
10 09 08 07 06 05 04 03 02 01

Printed and bound in Great Britain by
Creative Print and Design (Wales), Ebbw Vale

This text is dedicated to every nurse and midwife who has striven to improve their practice

Special Recognition

A special thanks is expressed to James Earl Cox for providing additional editorial support while this book was being written

In memory to the late
Lorna Elizabeth Haynes
(1963–1996)
Senior Sister and Emergency Nurse Practitioner
Accident and Emergency Services
Newham General Hospital

Contents

List of Tables

Foreword

Clinical effectiveness is a term used daily in health care in the UK particularly with the advent of *Clinical Governance*. For nursing, midwifery and health visiting it is an important concept that assures that patients receive appropriate clinical interventions, which either improve or maintain their health status or enable a dignified death. Clinically effective care also allows for patient choice in care and treatment and recognizes that what is provided has to be within the resources available.

The authors of this book have produced a seminal text that explores clinical effectiveness with regard to the role of the Clinical Nurse Specialist and Nurse Practitioner. In so doing they have articulated research findings through the use of case studies that clearly link theory to practice. The book's approach emphasizes the importance of using evidence based practice in day to day clinical activity and illustrates how the Clinical Nurse Specialist and Nurse Practitioner roles fit within the health care delivery system of the UK. The book demonstrates that these nurses and midwives are highly skilled; competent practitioners who have well-developed enhanced patient skills and care for patients and groups of patients in complex situations. They also act as a resource to many other clinicians and troubleshoot practice issues.

The framework used within the case studies is one that all Clinical Nurse Specialists and Nurse Practitioners can use to develop, compare and contrast their own roles. This book serves as an exceptional basis for informing health care organisations about how current roles may be reconstructed and new posts developed for essential and cost effective care. For the student it provides an opportunity to understand how clinically effective care is provided.

SUE NORMAN
Chief Executive/Registrar,
United Kingdom Central Council for Nursing,
Midwifery and Health Visiting London

Preface

This book represents the findings of a one and a half year study examining clinical effectiveness among clinical nurse specialists and nurse practitioners in England. The purpose of the text is to clarify what clinical effectiveness is and how it can be achieved. Key issues influencing practice have been brought to the fore and examined in the light of current evidence so that practice can be enhanced. The latest treatment modalities including medical, nursing and midwifery regimens are presented.

A special feature of this text is the presentation of research and case studies that illuminate evidence for the delivery of clinically effective care. Chapter 1 addresses clinical effectiveness, national guidelines for achieving clinically effective care, nursing diagnosis, roles associated with clinical nurse specialist and nurse practitioner practice, curriculum guidelines for advanced practice, competencies associated with clinical effectiveness, clinical supervision, clinical governance and shared governance. Chapter 2 presents the findings of a qualitative study that discerned factors that foster and hinder clinically effective care. The research questions, design and methods associated with exploratory, first level descriptive research are described and the findings illuminate today's dilemmas associated with achieving clinical effectiveness. The chapter concludes with recommendations for practice.

Chapter 3 reviews the findings of a follow on national study addressing clinical effectiveness and the realities of practice. The research questions, aims of the study, design and methods are described. Quantitative (Mann-Whitney U and Wilcoxin) data reveal significant correlations between the experiences of clinical nurse specialists and nurse practitioners in their drive to provide clinically effective care. Chapter 4 presents a case study associated with caring for the patient in septic shock. Management of the patient with multiple organ failure subsequent to sepsis is described within the context of critical care. Chapter 5 presents a case study associated with caring for the patient with tuberculosis. Transmission of the disease, drug resistance and side effects within the context of medical and nursing management are addressed.

Chapter 6 presents a case study associated with caring for the HIV positive pregnant woman. Implications for care of the woman, her partner, children and the newborn infant are explicated. Issues associated with confidentiality and trust are discussed within the context of modern healthcare delivery. Chapter 7 presents a case study associated with caring for the woman in obstetric crisis. Compounding factors include management and delivery of care in gestational diabetes mellitus, its causes in the Asian population and associated complications for the mother and infant. Chapter 8 presents a case study associated with promoting comfort for a patient suffering from cancer through the use of complementary therapies in conjunction with traditional Western orthodox medicine. The role of the clinical nurse specialist and nurse practitioner in relation to the use of complementary therapies is considered. The background to recommending complementary therapies in order to promote comfort is provided along with a review of various complementary therapies and their use in practice. Chapter 9 presents a case study associated with caring for the patient with leg ulcers. Special problems associated with the 'diabetic foot', neuropathy and peripheral vascular disease are considered.

The preliminary research for this book and development of its case studies took place at Newham Healthcare NHS Trust in London. Newham Healthcare NHS Trust is a 553-bedded Trust with healthcare facilities located at Newham General Hospital in Plaistow, St Andrews Hospital in Bow and the Shrewsbury Centre in Forest Gate. These facilities serve a population of approximately 280 000 people who live within the London Borough of Newham. This number may be higher due to refugees and migrants. An exact figure cannot be determined due to the transient nature of refugees and migrants.

In 1998 approval was given to the Trust to develop Newham General Hospital for acute and general services within this borough. Facilities provided by St Andrew's Hospital are to be transferred to Newham General Hospital following development of a new ambulatory care centre with 'walk in service' and health village. It is intended for approximately 25 per cent of local outpatients to be treated away from the main hospital site in community-based premises nearer to their own homes. As part of the Department of Health initiatives to improve health care, the Trust has developed a new admissions unit adjacent to Accident and Emergency and is improving services for children in Accident and Emergency by providing dedicated facilities for children separate from those used by adult patients at Newham General Hospital. In addition, improvements in intensive care and coronary care have led to the creation of a combined intensive therapy and high dependency unit and a separate coronary care unit.

Changing the way services are delivered to patients by ensuring the highest quality of expertise in nursing and midwifery care for inpatients and outpatients is regarded as the foundation of clinical effectiveness. Therefore, Newham Healthcare NHS Trust was regarded as an appropriate environment for researching clinical effectiveness. Newham Healthcare NHS Trust provides the following services in which nursing and midwifery care are provided:

- *Accident and Emergency Department* – provides a full range of 'front line' services and facilities that, are crucial to saving lives and supporting people in crisis.
- *Women's Health Services* – includes obstetrics, gynaecology, special baby care and IVF (in vitro fertilisation). These services are provided routinely through outpatient and inpatient services.

- *Medical Services and Elderly Services* – includes cardiology, diabetology, endocrinology, gastroenterology, haematology, respiratory medicine, dermatology, neurology, coronary care, HIV and AIDS, genito-urinary medicine and the acute care of the elderly.
- *Surgical Services* – includes the departments of anaesthetics, operating theatres and sterile supplies, intensive therapy, orthopaedics, surgery (including outpatient services), podiatry, ophthalmology, ENT, Day Care, and urology.

It is our intention for this text to be used as a reference when considering how clinically effective care can be achieved. It provides solid evidence and guidelines for practice. When these are utilised, practice will be enhanced and the practitioner will be making a difference in the delivery of care.

CAROL LYNN COX
ADRIAN REYES-HUGHES

List of Contributors

Sonya Ahluwalia, MSc., BSc. (Hons), RGN is Research Assistant at the City University, St Bartholomew School of Nursing and Midwifery, London.

Carol Lynn Cox, Ph.D., MSc., M.A. Ed., PG. Dip.Ed., BSc. (Hons), RGN is Professor of Advanced Clinical Practice at the City University, St Bartholomew School of Nursing and Midwifery, London and Consultant Nurse, Research and Education Related to Practice at the Newham Healthcare NHS Trust, London.

Virginia Gleissberg, MSc., BSc. (Hons), RGN is a TB Clinical Nurse Specialist at Newham Healthcare NHS Trust, London.

Rebecca Hall, BSc. (Hons), RGN is a TB Clinical Nurse Specialist at Newham Healthcare NHS Trust, London.

Joanne Hutchinson, BSc. (Hons), RM, RGN is Diabetic Midwife Specialist at Newham General Hospital, Plaistow, London.

Dawn Kavanagh, BSc. (Hons), Dip. Nursing, RGN is a Practice Development Nurse, Critical Care (Intensive Care and High Dependency Units) at Newham General Hospital, Plaistow, London.

Ann M. Price, BSc. (Hons), P.G.C.E., RGN is Lecturer-Practitioner, Intensive Care Unit at the Royal Free Hospital, Hampstead Health, London.

Adrian Reyes-Hughes, MSc., Dip. H.S.M., Dip.N. (London), RGN is Director of Policy and Standards, United Kingdom Central Council for Nursing, Midwifery and Health Visiting, London and Honorary Senior Lecturer, City University, St Bartholomew School of Nursing and Midwifery, London.

Judith Sunderland, BSc. (Hons), R.M., RGN is a HIV Specialist Midwife, Ante-Natal Clinic at Newham General Hospital, Plaistow, London.

Michael van Orsouw, RGN is a Vascular Nurse Practitioner at Newham General Hospital, Plaistow, London.

CHAPTER 1

Clinical Effectiveness, Nursing Diagnosis and the Role of the Clinical Nurse Specialist and Nurse Practitioner

CAROL LYNN COX, PH.D., MSc., MA ED., PG. DIP. ED., BSc. (HONS), RGN
AND SONYA AHLUWALIA, MSc., BSc. (HONS), RGN

Introduction

Clinical effectiveness has become the cornerstone and quintessence of the nursing profession and is the central focus for medicine and other allied professions. It has recently been acknowledged at the governmental level by establishing the National Centre for Clinical Excellence (Department of Health 1999a) and introducing clinical governance (Department of Health 1999b). Together these areas are involved in the government's ten-year modernisation strategy to ensure the delivery of high quality care across the National Health Service (NHS).

National standards of *good practice* are in the process of being evaluated in order to identify the efficiency and effectiveness of both existing and new interventions (Department of Health 1999a). Restructuring the NHS through the introduction of clinical governance initiatives has meant that clinical effectiveness becomes one of the key themes in the Department of Health's strategy for improving patient care (Department of Health 1998a).

As a concept, clinical effectiveness has been used as an umbrella for an array of terms that encompass: evidence based practice; outcomes research; clinical audit; and clinical governance. All these attempt to monitor the effectiveness of medical and nursing interventions in order to enhance the quality of patient care.

Clinical Effectiveness

Although various definitions of clinical effectiveness exist such as the Royal College of Nursing (1996) and National Health Service Executive (1996) definitions, the working definition this book has adopted is the widely cited definition of clinical effectiveness from the National Health Service Executive:

> Clinical Effectiveness is demonstrated when specific clinical interventions do what they are intended to do, which is to maintain and improve health whilst securing the greatest possible health gain from available resources. (NHSE 1996, p. 2)

Recent endeavours to modernise the NHS have led to clinical effectiveness initiatives that strive to provide high quality patient care that is both cost effective and based on the best evidence available. Modernising the NHS has included government initiatives set out in the following white papers: *New NHS Modern & Dependable Services* (Department of Health 1997), *A First Class Service: Quality in the New NHS* (Department of Health 1998b).

The introduction of clinical governance aims to provide a framework to continuously improve the quality of services in the NHS and safeguard the high standards of care by creating an environment in which excellence in clinical care can flourish (Department of Health 1998a).

Consequently clinical effectiveness is high on the political agenda and an area that will have important consequences for identifying the rational for patient care as well as focusing on each clinician's professional accountability to provide effective care. It is most certainly an area that cannot be ignored. The commission for health improvement will monitor the implementation of clinical governance initiatives across the NHS and undertake external clinical audits across NHS Trusts. Together these various strategies envisage a new and modern NHS that provides cost effective, clinically effective and high quality care to patients.

Providing effective nursing care to patients has been shown to be effective, efficient and cost effective and is a fundamental component of providing evidence based care. Interestingly, clinical effectiveness is not an unfamiliar concept to the nursing profession. It is an area that has been constantly addressed in relation to improving the effectiveness of nursing interventions and can be dated back to the pioneering work of Florence Nightingale. Over the last thirty years, the evaluation of particular nursing interventions, for example wound care management, management of pressure sores and the organisation of nursing care, has been scrutinised. The shift away from task orientated nursing care to patient focused care through primary nursing and the introduction of nursing development units is only one of many areas that have been undertaken in order to improve the efficiency of patient care.

Clinical effectiveness is an important area relevant to all aspects of patient care. The current climate of the NHS is one where economic rationalisation is a perpetual theme. By addressing clinical effectiveness, the care provided to patients is based on the knowledge that a particular intervention makes a difference to patient care and will, therefore, not only improve the efficiency and effectiveness of interventions but reduce the overall cost of unnecessary interventions. It makes sound economic sense. This has been highlighted in the literature, where it has been stipulated that if practice is evidence based it is more likely to be cost effective, appropriate and justifiable (Hicks 1997).

National Guidelines for Achieving Clinically Effective Care

The guidelines for developing clinical effectiveness were introduced in 1996 by the Royal College of Nursing (RCN 1996) and the National Health Service Executive (NHSE 1996). Their frameworks provided a step-by-step approach for individuals and organisations to use in order to provide nursing interventions that were based on existing research that demonstrated that a particular intervention improved the care of particular patient groups. These frameworks attempted to empower individuals to develop a climate conducive to providing nursing care that was based on the best evidence available.

There has been very little research into developing clinical effectiveness. Although there are guidelines and initiatives on developing clinical effectiveness (NHSE 1996; RCN 1996), there have been very few studies that specifically identify how clinical effectiveness is applied to directly influence practice (see for example, Dopson *et al* 1999, *Promoting Action on Clinical Effectiveness*). National databases have now been established across the United Kingdom in order to disseminate research findings on clinically effective care, such as the Cochrane Collaboration (International Database), Research and Development Units and The National Institute for Clinical Excellence (NICE).

Recent clinical effectiveness initiatives include the National Institute for Clinical Excellence (NICE) that provides guidelines for health professionals about the effectiveness of particular interventions for specific client groups. Most recently, the government launched its new initiatives on clinical governance (DoH 1999b), aiming to develop a working environment conducive to developing clinically effective care. However, it is also important and necessary to acknowledge how clinical effectiveness is applied in practice and to explore how this can be further used to enhance the quality of care provided to patients.

When entering the arena of clinical effectiveness it is necessary to ensure that the implementation of good practice is based on the best available evidence. What constitutes *good* evidence is controversial and involves the naturalistic versus the scientific debate. Do randomised controlled trials (RCTs) and quasi-experimental research (that is scientific research methodologies) provide more accurate, valid and reliable findings in comparison to the richness and subjectivity of qualitative research such as an individual's perceptions and life experiences? The scientific versus naturalistic inquiry is one area that remains frequently debated in the literature. This has contributed toward creating a hierarchy of *best evidence* where randomised controlled trials are considered to provide the best and most reliable evidence in comparison to qualitative analysis. It can only be postulated that each inquiry has its own individualistic value and that certain evaluations would be most suited to an RCT, for example clinical trials of drugs, the efficiency of various therapies, while other interventions would benefit from a qualitative inquiry, for example, the care of the dying patient using a grounded theory approach to understand the individual oncology patient's perceptions of dying. Triangulating the two approaches where appropriate can enhance the reliability and validity of the research findings. This will be a debate that will continue for some time to come.

Nursing Diagnosis

Nursing diagnosis is derived from an assessment of the client. It is a statement about the actual or potential health status of the client explicated in nursing language/terminology. Abdellah and Levine indicated the need to specialise nursing's language as early as 1965 when they described nursing diagnosis. They stated in their seminal text on nursing practice that:

> Crucial to the development of nursing science is the nurse's ability to make a nursing diagnosis and prescribe nursing actions that will result in specific responses in the client. Nursing diagnosis is a determination of the nature and extent of nursing problems presented by individual clients or families receiving nursing care. The position is taken that it is an independent function of the professional nurse to make a nursing diagnosis and to decide upon a course of action to be followed for the solution of the problem. (Abdellah and Levine 1965:25)

It was recognised that nurses share a common language in relation to some client problems with other disciplines such as medicine and physiotherapy. However there are some unique differences in aspects of practice amongst the disciplines and, over time it has become recognized that nursing also has a unique language that is shared within nursing specialities. For this reason in 1973 the first Conference for the Classification of Nursing Diagnosis convened (Carpenito 1997) and the process of developing a taxonomy of nursing diagnosis began. Today, the North American Nursing Diagnosis Association (NANDA 1992) nursing diagnosis classification and taxonomies are accepted as the international standard of nursing diagnoses. Each nursing diagnostic group, 123 NANDA-approved diagnoses, with definitions of the problem, defining characteristics or risk factors and related factors are described in Carpenito's (1997) text and can be used by nurse specialists to communicate the special needs of the client to other nurses. In many nursing education programmes in the United Kingdom and on the continent of Europe interest in nursing diagnosis is increasing. The NANDA-approved diagnoses have been incorporated into foundation programmes where the nursing process is taught.

Carpenito (1997) has indicated that it is important for the client and the client's family to understand and agree the nursing diagnosis as well as nursing goals and interventions planned in association with the diagnosis. Therefore, the nurse should indicate to the client and the client's family that nursing diagnosis terminology is designed to give nurses consistent language for communicating information about the client across nursing specialties. By the diagnosis being described in an internationally accepted language, this means that the diagnosis will be understood along with its prescribed nursing goals and interventions among nurses around the world. This is an important reason for explicating a nursing diagnosis whenever client health needs or problems are identified. It is critical, however that nurses keep in mind that, regardless of the nursing terminology used, all explanations given to the client and the client's family must be given within the context of their cultural background, educational level and ability to understand the nursing care regimen prescribed.

Nursing diagnosis is integrated with the nursing process. There is a cyclic relationship between the steps of the nursing process, nursing diagnosis and associated nursing goals and interventions. Each step within the nursing process depends on the accuracy of the step preceding it (Carpenito 1997; Gordon 1987). Although in reality the steps of the nursing process are continuous and interrelated, the steps of assessing, diagnosing, planning, implementing and evaluating are dependent upon the clinical expertise of the nurse and the knowledge the nurse has that underpins that expertise. Nursing diagnosis is an integral function of nursing practice delineated in the North American Nurse Practitioner Faculty Curriculum Guidelines (NONPF 1995). Nurse specialists, be they clinical nurse specialists or nurse practitioners, collect data to determine the need for nursing care and to assist other healthcare practitioners in determining the healthcare needs of the client. In order to effectively exchange data about the client, nurse specialists should consciously integrate nursing diagnosis into their utilization of the nursing process. This will enhance the clinical effectiveness of care as well as the quality of care that clients receive.

Roles Associated with Clinical Nurse Specialists and Nurse Practitioners

Highly experienced nurses with an in-depth knowledge base of a particular speciality have become common in the acute care and primary care sector. Expert nurses who have extensive clinical expertise, knowledge and skills have been found to provide a higher quality of nursing care (Benner 1984; Benner and Tanner 1987; Benner and Wrubel 1989). The nursing care provided by Clinical Nurse Specialists and Nurse Practitioners has been highlighted as making a difference to patient care (Brykczynski 1989; Fenton and Brykczynski 1993; Walsh *et al.* 1999). The care provided to patients has been found to be of a higher quality in comparison to nursing care provided by less experienced and knowledgeable nurses (Benner 1984; Brykczynski 1989; Fenton and Brykczynski 1993).

Although there are differences between the role of the Nurse Practitioner (NP) and the role of the Clinical Nurse Specialist (CNS), they are both considered to be experts in their specialist fields. Nurse Practitioners are pushing hard at the traditional boundaries of practice and are frequently involved in task-orientated care that overlaps with medical interventions (Walsh *et al.* 1999). Their role has been associated with the reduction in junior doctors' working hours and is often associated with tasks normally carried out by junior doctors, for example, intravenous cannulation, drawing blood for arterial blood analysis and physical assessment. Nurse Practitioners work in the secondary (acute) and primary (community) care sectors and frequently may be seen working in outpatient clinics, accident and emergency, orthopaedics, medicine, surgery and general practice.

Clinical Nurse Specialists remain more actively involved in the care of hospitalised patients, although these nurses too are found in the patient clinic environment. The most common fields of care for Clinical Nurse Specialists exist in diabetes, palliative care and continence nursing (McGee *et al.* 1996). The multi-faceted roles that are most commonly associated with the CNS role include: educator, researcher, consultant, expert practitioner and change agent (Hamric and Spross 1989; Miller 1995; Schneider 1992; Vitello-Cicciu 1984). Other roles that have been highlighted include the role of the CNS as an entrepreneur and collaborator (Hazeleton 1993) and as a caretaker, (Schaefer 1992). A Delphi Study of expert nurse practice identified an additional 13 characteristics that were demonstrated amongst expert practitioners in nursing, health visiting and midwifery (Butterworth and Bishop 1995). The study findings highlighted that the quality of patient care was improved. This related to CNS involvement in standard setting and also emphasized how expert practitioners provided a supportive learning environment for their colleagues' professional development.

Although both similarities and differences exist amongst these roles (Fenton 1985), both roles have been identified as providing high quality nursing care

(Chuk 1997). Therefore, these multifaceted roles place the CNS and NP in an ideal position to develop clinically effective care.

The National Organisation of Nurse Practitioners Faculties Curriculum Guidelines

The National Organisation of Nurse Practitioners Faculties (NONPF 1995) developed a competency framework that can be implemented in order to achieve clinically effective care. There are six domains of Advanced Nursing Practice identified in this framework that have been drawn from extensive research conducted by Fenton (1985), Brykczynski (1989) and Benner (1984). Their research involved observations of practice and interviews with both clinical nurse specialists and nurse practitioners in North America. The six domains are:

Management of Client Health/Illness Status

Examples include:
1. Health Promotion/Disease Prevention including providing anticipatory guidance and counselling regarding wellness, lifestyle, disease risks, and potential changes in health status.
2. Developing and analysing appropriate differential diagnoses for presenting client symptoms.

The Nurse–Client Relationship

Examples include:
1. Creating a relationship that acknowledges the client's strengths and assisting the client in addressing his/her health needs.
2. Providing emotional and informational support to clients and their families.

The Teaching–Coaching Function

Examples include:
1. Creating an environment in which effective learning can take place and specifically altering the environment if necessary so that the client can attend to the learning process.
2. Monitoring the client's behaviour and delineating outcomes of learning as a useful guide to evaluating the effectiveness of care and the need to change or maintain teaching strategies.

Professional Role

Examples include:

1. Functioning in a variety of role dimensions: healthcare provider, consultant, educator, administrator and researcher.
2. Evaluating the implications of contemporary health policy for healthcare providers and consumers.

Managing and Negotiating Health Care Delivery Systems

Examples include:

1. Providing care for individuals, families; and communities within integrated healthcare services using nationally accepted guidelines and standards.
2. Negotiation which includes assessment, planning, implementation and evaluation of healthcare delivery collaboratively with other healthcare professionals, using approaches that recognise each one's expertise and interest to meet the comprehensive needs of clients.

Monitoring and Ensuring the Quality of Healthcare Practices

Examples include:

1. Critically evaluating and applying research studies pertinent to client care management and outcomes.
2. Monitoring peers, self and delivery systems through quality assurance activities and total quality management as part of continuous quality improvement.

This framework is used as a practice based assessment tool for the Masters in Advanced Nursing Practice in North America. It has also been used as the basis for constructing the case studies in this textbook in order to demonstrate how clinically effective nursing care is achieved among clinical nurse specialists and nurse practitioners at the Newham Healthcare Trust.

Clinical Supervision

Clinical supervision has been identified as an important facet for promoting and enhancing practice through reflection (Winstanley 1999). In 1997 the Department of Health published its perspective on modernising healthcare delivery (DoH 1997). In this document, it indicates that one aspect of modernisation within nursing services is the introduction of clinical supervision. The Department of Health (1997) identifies clinical supervision as a term used to describe a formal process of professional support and learning which enables individual practitioners to develop knowledge and competence, assume responsibility for their own practice and enhance patient care in complex clinical situations. Faugier (1992) suggests clinical supervision should be about empowerment, not control, and that the route to professional accountability is through the building of confidence and self-esteem. Clinical supervision should enable nurses to be able to:

1. Reflect on their feelings and attitudes towards care given to clients and their families.
2. Be clear about issues presented by the client and related legislative care.
3. Be clear about the client's healthcare needs and how to manage these.
4. Write an action plan of care for the client and the client's family.
5. Record the action plan of care in a professional record.
6. Maintain good practice and feel supported in that practice.

Therefore, the following becomes essential in relation to nursing practice:

1. Recognition of the importance of enhancing practice through reflection.
2. Knowledge of physical, emotional and behavioural signs and predisposing factors of health and illness and how care is managed.
3. Identification of roles and responsibilities of nursing staff in relation to assuming functions associated with clinical supervision.
4. Interdisciplinary engagement in clinical supervision.
5. Record keeping in relation to practice and clinical supervision.
6. Working collaboratively with the interdisciplinary healthcare team.
7. Knowledge of mechanisms available for obtaining professional advice and guidance.

The United Kingdom Central Council for Nursing, Midwifery and Health Visiting indicates that clinical supervision assists practitioners to develop their skills, knowledge and professional values throughout their careers. As such it enables practitioners to develop a deeper understanding of what it is to be an accountable practitioner, and to link this to the reality of practice more easily than has been previously possible (UKCC 1996).

Clinical supervision is regarded as an essential part of nursing practice. Clinical supervision focuses its lens clearly on clinical practice, which is how practitioners engage with clients for the benefit of improving care and standards of care, as well as developing personal and professional skills and satisfaction in nursing. Individuals who choose to become supervisors within the clinical supervision process should be fully trained in clinical supervision techniques.

Clinical Governance

The National Health Service (NHS) has been providing integrated healthcare services for patients since 1948 (DoH 2000a). Over this time the service has evolved and has been a substantial partner with the government in introducing reforms intended to improve healthcare delivery and the management of resources. The government has restated its aim to develop a NHS in which all patients have fair access to consistently high quality healthcare. The emphasis on high quality is a central component of the Government's plan (DoH 1997; 1998; 1999a; 1999b; 2000a; 2000b) for modernisation of the health service. The plan has led to the establishment of a number of complementary processes for ensuring continuous improvement in healthcare delivery at both the local and national level. The term clinical governance has been coined to describe the overall process of which clinical effectiveness is a central component. It is the first quality initiative to be underpinned by legislation (1999 Health Act).

Clinical governance should be seen as a process of introducing health improvement measures over time which are capable of responding to change brought on by developments in science, medicine, nursing, midwifery, management and healthcare resourcing. NHS facilities must develop a culture of innovation, enterprise, efficiency and good customer services in order to create and sustain clinical governance arrangements. Changes in local health services should mirror changes which occurr in national exemplar services. Clinical governance demonstrates responsiveness to patient need and demand and continuously ensures the best possible clinical and health outcomes for patients and their families.

Clinical governance can be defined as

> a framework through which the NHS organisations are accountable for continuously improving the quality of their services and safeguarding high standards of care by creating an environment in which clinical excellence in clinical care will flourish (DoH 1998:33).

It is a vital ingredient that will enable healthcare facilities to achieve a service in which quality of health care is paramount. It may be considered to be corporate responsibility for clinical performance, and although it does not replace professional self-regulation and individual clinical judgement in practice, it adds an extra dimension that provides the public with guarantees about standards of clinical care.

Developing Tools for Quality

The delivery of a dependable and high quality healthcare system depends on the production of clearly described standards of care, means of achievement and clinical outcomes. The processes for reaching the standards must be well understood by all people involved in healthcare delivery. Standards are set in a variety of ways within the NHS. Those most visible are:

- Professional and statutory bodies like the United Kingdom Central Council for Nursing, Midwifery and Health Visiting
- Schools of medicine, nursing and midwifery
- Research and development output
- National machinery
- Local machinery
- Voluntary organisations and user groups.

Much of the variation in health status across patient populations is recognized as the result of differing socio-economic status within populations. Access to healthcare resources also varies according to geography, tradition and economics and will influence the determination of local standards and performance in healthcare services. Every healthcare organisation has a duty to ensure that its standards of care match those in the best performing organisations according to the Department of Health (DoH 1998a; 1999a). A key to the delivery of effective clinical governance is for healthcare facilities to become *learning* organisations where examples of good practice are rapidly incorporated into everyday work and a spirit of innovation, enterprise and patient centred approaches are employed throughout individual organisations.

In the Government's White Paper *The New NHS: Modern and Dependable* (DoH 1997) some of the aspects of cultural change that are required at the local level were defined. It is clear that professional and statutory bodies have a vital role to play in setting and promoting standards of care. These organisations emphasize quality. This, therefore, requires healthcare practitioners to accept responsibility for developing and maintaining standards within their local NHS organisations. Quality is seen as central to clinical governance and Within that framework there is an expectation that all healthcare professionals will see the concepts of clinical governance as part of their responsibility within the organisations in which they work.

Standard Setting

Standard setting is informed nationally and locally by National Service Frameworks. The art and science of medical care remains the cornerstone of clinical encounters with patients. The form of clinical encounters has been identified as infinitely variable and difficult to define (Gutteridge 2000). It is within this context that the government has set out an approach to matching consistency in quality across the NHS with sensitivity to the needs of individual patients seeking care within their local community. A new model is emerging which requires considerable development at the local level. All attempts to promote local clinical judgement should be informed by evidence based clinical standards.

National standards are set through National Service Frameworks that define generic and specific clinical standards for a range of services and conditions. In all parts of the country, the NHS is required to organise its services to match the standards set in the frameworks and to ensure equity in provision and access. National standards that have been set are reviewed through the National Institute for Clinical Excellence (NICE). This Institute assesses the clinical effectiveness of a wide range of current and proposed clinical interventions including drug therapies, surgical procedures and clinical devices. Assessments are made within the context of cost effectiveness and clinical effectiveness.

Individual healthcare facilities are required to develop local mechanisms for setting clinical and service standards within the context of their own clinical governance structures and processes. A board associated with each healthcare facility is required to ensure that service groups are properly supported in developing standards for patients and their relatives in relation to healthcare provision. It is at this critical interface that healthcare facilities must involve patients, families and the voluntary sector in the process of defining relevant and achievable standards of care that take into account local conditions. Clinical governance transforms modern management concepts of corporate governance and introduces concepts of the therapeutic process in order to ensure continuous quality improvement. Lifelong learning is integral to clinical governance. The concepts of lifelong learning, integrated into healthcare facilities, give all NHS staff the knowledge and the tools with which to offer the most modern, effective and high quality care to patients and their families.

Responsibility for Ensuring High Quality Care

The responsibility for ensuring high quality care has been, in the past, defined by individual healthcare professionals. This principle is enshrined in the Hippocratic oath and was developed by the health boards of Renaissance Italy, the Royal Colleges in this country and over time by national registration systems for doctors, nurses, midwives and other healthcare professionals. These systems have emphasized the need for ensuring effective education and training and for regular review of performance. The General Medical Council and the United Kingdom Central Council for Nursing, Midwifery and Health Visiting (UKCC 1992a; 1992b; 1998) have set out in their documents what doctors, nurses and midwives must do:

be professionally competent
perform consistently well

practice ethically
do patients no harm
be an effective team player
take action when poor practice places patients at risk
provide care that is safe, supportive and free from abuse.

Components of Clinical Governance

Clinical governance is based on continuing professional development (lifelong learning), risk management and clinical effectiveness. These three areas of activity include a wide variety of functions and must be actively supported by integrating information and human resource systems. Within this context five themes within clinical governance require attention. These are:

national consistency
accountability
quality assurance improvement
management of poor performance
collaboration and teamwork.

All of the aforementioned can be managed under organisational frameworks designed to address clinical effectiveness, clinical risk management, non-clinical risk management, performance monitoring, and staff and organisational development. The critical component within this is that all healthcare practitioners must recognize their place within clinical governance and practice according to standards that have been developed to ensure the provision of high quality care.

Shared Governance – A Model of Nursing and Midwifery Service

Shared governance is recognized internationally as a tool directed towards facilitating the maturation of the nurse and midwife professional (Porter-O'Grady 1994). It is a creative approach to professional accountability that has its roots embedded in clinical effectiveness, clinical supervision and clinical governance. In 1984 Timothy Porter-O'Grady and Sharon Finnigan published their seminal text *Shared Governance for Nursing* (Porter-O'Grady and Finnigan 1984). Donaho (1984:ix) indicated in the Foreword to Porter-O'Grady's and Finnigan's text that

> Today's professional nurse values competency. Included within this value is the desire to assume accountability, to clearly articulate what nursing practice

entails, define excellence in that practice, and determine, through evaluation, the quality of care provided, as well as the competence of the practitioner.

Although written nearly two decades ago, the words reflect the perspective of nursing and midwifery today and are seen to be central to the platform of shared governance.

Nurses and midwives work within the contexts of primary, secondary and tertiary care. The challenge within all of these contexts is to facilitate a process of professional governance within what appears to be primarily centralised hierarchical structures. This requires a clear understanding of what professional governance is about and integrated support systems that achieve the principles of professional accountability in practice. According to Donaho (Porter-O'Grady and Finnigan 1984) and Porter-O'Grady (1994) it requires valuing a decentralised approach to governance and management which allows for professionals to maintain as much influence as possible about decisions related to clinical practice, the environment in which work takes place, professional development and personal fulfilment.

This does not mean that decentralisation is a requirement for shared governance to flourish. Indeed, within centralised structures the principles of decentralisation can come to the fore through implementation of a shared governance model. A shared governance model creates a professional work environment that reflects a higher level of accountability in patient care. Within the model, all nurses and midwives have a stake in their workplace and its practice activities. Therefore, clinical practice, levels of job satisfaction and productivity are increased. According to Porter-O'Grady and Finnigan (1984) through the model, nurses and midwives can become truly professional, with all of the status, opportunities and values that professionalism implies.

The NHS is at a crossroads in relation to its modernisation goals. Changes in its healthcare delivery system are having a substantial impact on all of its healthcare professionals. Nursing and midwifery are being affected greatly by these changes as expectations associated with clinical governance mandate changes in practice, professional accountability and self-governance. It is recognised, particularly within the current climate of nursing and midwifery staff shortages that there is:

- an increasing economic value of nurses and midwives;
- a requirement to create a workplace in which healthcare provision is satisfying and rewarding;
- a need to increase participation of nurses and midwives in decisions that affect their practice and profession.

All of the aforementioned can be recognized and implemented effectively within a shared governance model. Within the framework, the professional character of the participants is reflected, positive behaviours and practices are promoted and systems are enhanced that provide ongoing support for the professional role of nurses and midwives in the provision of healthcare services.

A Model of Service

The creation of a healthcare organisation that fits the purposes of the NHS Plan (DoH 2000a) is challenging. Making nursing and midwifery practice visible within the structural design of the organisation further complicates the process of planning. Assessing the healthcare organisation and encouraging its movement toward democratic and rational approaches to management of human resources and practice are common themes in management theory. Considerable work has been undertaken to bring the management of human resources to a realistic and practical level where alternative structures that foster the therapeutic process and decision-making at the lowest possible level in the organisation occur (DoH 1999a, 2000a, 2000b). This is at the core of shared governance in nursing and midwifery services and mirrors the initiatives delineated through clinical governance to ensure continuous quality improvement and high quality care.

Continuous quality improvement and the delivery of high quality care in nursing and midwifery services are dependent upon effective co-ordination and integration of professional behaviour, accountability and clinical practice. This is significant since all elements within the healthcare delivery system are interdependent. Collective interaction influences the outcome of patient and family care. According to Porter-O'Grady (1991) this process is highly complex. It recognizes that each unit of activity depends on others for the fulfilment of the goals of the entire organisation.

Professional Accountability and Clinical Practice

In order for nurses and midwives to be truly accountable within their scope of professional practice, they must be given the authority and the autonomy to make decisions and control over the implementation and outcome of the decisions. Without these conditions, accountability cannot be taken forward and *becomes an empty phrase* (Porter-O'Grady 1991:459). Shared governance transforms the way the healthcare organisation provides for participation in and ownership of service provision. Nurses and midwives at every level within the organisation are recognised as playing an integral role in decision-making that affects activity throughout the organisation. Governance is at the core of the system and authority and accountability are shared between and among the nursing and midwifery staff. The emphasis is on nurses and midwives entering into a partnership with other members of the multidisciplinary team that agree to meet the mission and objectives of the organisation and to fulfil the mandates of their profession and the government plans for continuous quality improvement. This is accomplished through the establishment of councils that control the practice, quality of care, continuing professional development and management of nursing and midwifery staff. The councils are staff nurse and midwife led and assert the following basic tenets:

- Nursing and midwifery practice is controlled by the staff. Issues that relate to practice originate and end with the staff. Shared governance standards have mechanisms that ensure staff accountability for the issues of practice that affect their discipline wherever they originate in the healthcare organisation.
- Continuous quality improvement is a staff issue. All quality improvement processes and initiatives must reflect staff ownership and staff must be able to operate effectively without management control or intervention within these. Porter-O'Grady (1991) indicates that quality includes control of staff access to and exit from the organisation and, therefore, includes review of staff credentials and staff privileges.
- Staff competence is dependent upon continuing professional development. It is recognised that this is not just the obligation of the healthcare organisation. It is a requirement of professional practice. As such it is the obligation of every practicing nurse and midwife to ensure that they are competent. Teaching and learning associated with continuing professional development must originate and be controlled by the staff. There is a mechanism maintained by the staff to demonstrate evidence of their continuing professional development to peers, other healthcare professionals, patients and their families.
- Management strategies that support staff roles are transparent. The decision regarding staff roles that fall within the auspices of the staff and managers at all levels within the organisation must be able to support the staff in the roles they undertake. Within this context, managers change from working within functional roles that relate to only their professional boundaries to roles that involve supporting the entire system. The manager becomes a resource person as the staff's role in the delivery of care and governance is redefined and developed. The manager becomes accountable for ensuring that support and resources are available to ensure that the staff can operate effectively in the delivery of high quality care.
- An integrating (co-ordinating) council '...pulls the components of the organisation together to provide consistency, communication, problem solving, decision making and relationships necessary to make the system work effectively.' (Porter-O'Grady 1991:462). All levels within the organisation are addressed in this integrating structure. Subsequently this ensures that a defined role for each type of practitioner, staff nurse, midwife or manager is understood and communicated throughout the organisation.

Shared governance is dependent upon the appropriate fulfilment of the obligations of all roles within the nursing and midwifery service. Through implementation of the model's councils and assumption of accountability a programme of continuous quality improvement evolves and the provision of quality health care is enhanced; the mission of the organisation can be successfully achieved. Key within this is the commitment of nursing and midwifery leadership at the outset and that the process of developing a shared governance model of service is taken forward by the staff.

Conclusion

This chapter has described clinical effectiveness, the national guidelines for achieving clinically effective care, nursing diagnosis, roles associated with clinical nurse specialist and nurse practitioner practice, the National Organisation of Nurse Practitioner Faculty competencies associated with advanced practice, clinical supervision and the constructs associated with clinical governance and shared governance. It has demonstrated that integration of these strategies and governance structures may be used as a mechanism for ensuring professional accountability, self-regulation of practice, continuous professional development and continuous quality improvement. These lead to the provision of high quality care. When developed as an integrated model for nursing and midwifery service it has much to contribute to the job satisfaction of nurses and midwives while taking forward the Government's agenda for the delivery of high quality patient care.

In Chapters 2 and 3 of this book, the findings of an exploratory study, which aimed to discover how clinically effective nursing care is fostered amongst Clinical Nurse Specialists (CNSs) and Nurse Practitioners (NPs), is described. Chapter 2 describes the qualitative component of the project and makes recommendations for practice enhancement. Chapter 3 describes the quantitative component of the project which aimed to discern whether the findings from the qualitative component could be substantiated nationally among a convenience sample of Clinical Nurse Specialists (CNSs) and Nurse Practitioners (NPs) who work the in the National Health Service (NHS) and private healthcare facilities.

References

Abdellah, F. and M. Levine (1965) *Better Patient Care Through Nursing Research*, New York, Macmillan

Benner, P. (1984) *From Novice to Expert: Excellence and Power in Clinical Nursing Practice*, Menlo Park, CA, Addison-Wesley

Brykczynski, K. A. (1989) 'An Interpretive Study Describing the Clinical Judgment of Nurse Practitioners', *Scholarly Inquiry for Nursing Practice: An Interpretive Journal*, 3(2), pp. 113–20

Butterworth, T. and V. Bishop (1995) 'Identifying the Characteristics of Optimum Practice: findings from a survey of practice experts in nursing, midwifery and health visiting', *Journal of Advanced Nursing*, 22(1), pp. 24–32

Carpenito, L. (1997) *Nursing Diagnosis Application to Clinical Practice*, 7th edn, New York, Lippincott

Chuk, P. (1997) 'Clinical Nurse Specialists and Quality Patient Care', *Journal of Advanced Nursing*, 26(3), pp. 501–6

Department of Health (1997) *The New NHS Modern and Dependable*, London, HMSO

Department of Health (1998a) *A First Class Service: Quality in the New NHS*, London, HMSO

Department of Health (1998b) *Saving Lives: Our Healthier Nation*, London, HMSO

Department of Health (1999a) *National Institute for Clinical Excellence*, London, HMSO

Department of Health (1999b) *Clinical Governance: Quality in the New NHS*, Leeds, NHSE

Department of Health (2000a) *The NHS Plan: A plan for investment, A plan for reform*, Norwich, HMSO

Department of Health (2000b) *The NHS Plan: the Government's Response to the Royal Commission on Long Term Care*, Norwich, HMSO

Donaho, B. (1984) Foreword in T. Porter-O'Grady and S. Finnigan (eds) *Shared Governance For Nursing*, Rockville and Royal Tunbridge Wells, Aspen Publication, Aspen Systems Corporation

Dopson, S., J. Gabbay, J. Locock and D. Chambers (1999) *Evaluation of the PACE Programme: final report*, Oxford Health Care Management Institute, Templeton College, University of Oxford, Wessex Institute for Health Research and Development, University of Southampton

Faugier, J. (1992) 'The Supervisory Relationship', in T. Butterworth and J. Faugier (eds), *Clinical Supervision and Mentorship in Nursing*, London, Chapman Hall

Fenton, M. (1985) 'Identifying Competencies of Clinical Nurse Specialists', *Journal of Nursing Administration*, 15(12), pp. 16–20

Fenton, M. and Brykczynski, K. (1993) 'Qualitative Distinctions and Similarities in the Practice of Clinical Nurse Specialists and Nurse Practitioners', *Journal of Professional Nursing*, 9(6), pp. 313–26

Gordon, M. (1987) *Nursing Diagnosis: Process and Application*, 2 edn, New York, McGraw-Hill

Gutteridge, C. (2000) *Newham Healthcare NHS Trust Clinical Governance Strategic Plan*, Plaistow, Newham Healthcare NHS Trust

Hamric, A. and J. Spross (1989) *The Clinical Nurse Specialist in Theory and Practice*, Philadelphia, W.B. Saunders

Hazeleton, J. (1993) 'Clinical Nurse Specialist Subroles: foundations for entrepreneurship', *Clinical Nurse Specialist*, 7(1), pp. 40–5

Hicks, C. (1997) 'Research: the Dilemma of Incorporating Research into Clinical Practice', *British Journal of Nursing*, 6(9), pp. 511–15

McGee, P., G. Casteldine and R. Brown (1996) 'A Survey of Specialist and Advanced Nursing Practice in England', *British Journal of Nursing*, 5(11), pp. 683–6

Miller, S. (1995) 'The Clinical Nurse Specialist: a way forward?' *Journal of Advanced Nursing*, 22(3), pp. 494–501

National Health Service Executive (1996) *Achieving Effective Practice: A clinical effectiveness and research information pack for nurses, midwives and health visitors*, Leeds, NHSE

NONPF National Organisation of Nurse Practitioners Faculties Curriculum Guidelines Task Force (1995) *Advanced Nursing Practice, Curriculum Guidelines and Programme Standards for Nurse Practitioner Education*, California

North American Nursing Diagnosis Association (1992) *Taxonomy of nursing diagnosis*, Philadelphia

Porter-O'Grady, T. (1991) 'Shared Governance for Nursing, Part 1: Creating the New Organisation', *AORN Journal*, 53(2), pp. 458–66

Porter-O'Grady, T. (1994) 'Whole Systems Shared Governance: Creating the Seamless Organisation', *Nursing Economics*, 12(4), pp. 187–95

Porter-O'Grady, T. and Finnigan, S. (1984) *Shared Governance For Nursing*, Rockville and Royal Tunbridge Wells, Aspen Publication, Aspen Systems Corporation

Royal College of Nursing (1996) *Clinical Effectiveness, A Royal College of Nursing Guide*, London, Royal College of Nursing

Schaefer, K. (1991) 'Taking Care of the Caretakers: a partial explanation of clinical nurse specialist practice', *Journal of Advanced Nursing*, 16(3), pp. 270–6

Schneider, J. (1992) 'Clinical Nurse Specialist; Role Definition as Discharge Planning Co-ordinator', *Clinical Nurse Specialist*, 6(1), pp. 36–39

UKCC (1992a) *Code of Professional Conduct*, London, United Kingdom Central Council for Nursing, Midwifery and Health Visiting

UKCC (1992b) *The Scope of Professional Practice*, London, United Kingdom Central Council for Nursing, Midwifery and Health Visiting

UKCC (1996) *Position Statement on Clinical Supervision for Nursing*, Midwifery and Health Visiting, London, United Kingdom Central Council

UKCC (1998) *Midwives Rules and Code of Practice*, London, United Kingdom Central Council for Nursing, Midwifery and Health Visiting

Vitello-Cicciu, J. (1984) 'Excellence in Critical Care: educating the clinical specialists', *Critical Care Quarterly*, 7(1) pp. 26–32

Walsh, M., A. Crumbie and S. Reveley (1999) *Nurse Practitioners Clinical Skills and Professional Issues*, Oxford, Butterworth Heinemann

Winstanley, J. (1999) *Evaluation of the efficacy of clinical supervision*, Nursing Times Monographs, No. 26

CHAPTER 2

Factors that Foster and Hinder Clinically Effective Care of Clinical Nurse Specialists and Nurse Practitioners: a Qualitative Study

CAROL LYNN COX AND SONYA AHLUWALIA

Introduction

This chapter describes the findings of an exploratory study that aimed to discover how clinically effective nursing care is fostered among Clinical Nurse Specialists (CNSs) and Nurse Practitioners (NPs) in a National Health Service (NHS) Trust in East London and makes recommendations for practice enhancement. The study was funded by the Central and East London Education Consortium (CELEC) and commenced in January 1999.

Multi-method technique was used to discern how clinically effective care is fostered among Clinical Nurse Specialists and Nurse Practitioners in the Trust. Qualitative approaches included non-participant observation of practice, discussions during observation and focus group meetings. Findings from the research identify areas that foster and hinder the ability of the Clinical Nurse Specialist and Nurse Practitioner to engage in and provide clinically effective nursing care.

Research Question and Aim and Objectives of the Study

The question that initiated the study was 'how is clinically effective care amongst Clinical Nurse Specialists and Nurse Practitioners at the Trust fostered?' The aim of the research was to explore how clinical effectiveness initiatives were developed among expert nurses designated as CNSs and NPs. In order to appreciate how such a complex phenomenon is understood, it was

necessary to find out how participants applied this concept in practice. Observations of clinical practice provided an insight into how clinical effectiveness was applied in practice. Informal discussions and focus group meetings provided an opportunity to explore issues and address rigour in qualitative research by providing participants with the opportunity to discuss and confirm the preliminary findings of the research.
Objectives of the research:

- identify current levels of clinical effectiveness amongst CNSs and NPs at the Trust;
- identify how clinically effective care is achieved among CNSs and NPs at the Trust;
- identify the competencies associated with clinically effective care at the Trust;
- determine levels of practice, which could be assumed by CNSs and NPs at the Trust;
- provide recommendations for improving clinically effective care among CNSs and NPs at the Trust;
- recommend avenues of study/preparation for assumption of extended practice roles.

Review of the Literature and Rationale for the Study

The NHS acts within a climate of economic rationalisation, efficiency and effectiveness. Therefore, providing clinically effective care to patients is high on the health care agenda. Recent endeavours to modernise the NHS have led to initiatives that strive to provide high quality patient care that is both cost effective and based on the best evidence available. Modernising the NHS has included government initiatives set out by the white papers: *New NHS Modern and Dependable Services* (Department of Health 1997) and *A First Class Service: Quality in the New NHS* (Department of Health 1998). These documents identify the provision of effective nursing care to patients is essential. Nursing care should be evidence based, efficient and cost effective. It has also been highlighted, in other publications, if practice is evidence based it is more likely to be cost effective, appropriate and justifiable (Hicks 1997).

The recent introduction of clinical governance aims to provide a framework to continuously improve the quality of services in the NHS and safeguard high standards of care by creating an environment in which excellence in clinical care can flourish (Department of Health 1999a). Consequently clinical effectiveness is an area that will have important implications for patient care as well as individual staff development. It is certainly an area that cannot be ignored.

There has been little research in the area of developing clinical effectiveness. However there are initiatives and guidelines that have been produced on developing clinical effectiveness (National Health Service Executive 1996; Royal College of Nursing 1996). Although guidelines are published, few studies specifically identify how clinical effectiveness is applied to directly influence practice (Dopson *et al.* 1999).

Recent clinical effectiveness initiatives include the National Institute for Clinical Excellence (Department of Health 1999b) that provides guidelines for health professionals about the effectiveness of particular interventions for specific patients. Most recently, the government launched its new initiatives on clinical governance, aiming to develop a working environment conducive to developing clinically effective care. It is necessary now to research how this concept is applied in practice and identify how this can be further used to enhance the quality of care provided to patients.

Guidelines for developing clinical effectiveness were introduced in 1996 by the Royal College of Nursing (RCN 1996) and the National Health Service Executive (NHSE 1996). Their frameworks provide a step-by-step approach to utilizing the research process and encourage individuals to develop a climate conducive to providing effective and efficient nursing care that is based on the best evidence available. What constitutes *good* evidence is a controversial area that encompasses the arena of randomised controlled trials, scientific enquiry and the naturalistic debate relating to qualitative research methodologies. Government initiatives in this field include the National Centre for Clinical Excellence (NICE) and more recently, initiation of clinical governance (Department of Health 1999a) where clinical effectiveness is one of the key themes.

Clinical effectiveness acts as an umbrella for an array of terms such as evidence based practice, clinical audits and outcomes research. Although various definitions of clinical effectiveness exist, the working definition for the research project described in this chapter has adopted the widely cited definition of clinical effectiveness from the National Health Service Executive (1996):

> Clinical Effectiveness is demonstrated when specific clinical interventions do what they are intended to do, which is to maintain and improve health whilst securing the greatest possible health gain from available resources. (NHSE 1996, p. 2)

Expert nurses who have extensive clinical expertise, knowledge and skills have been found to provide a higher quality of nursing care (Benner 1984; Benner and Tanner 1987). The nursing care provided by clinical nurse specialists and nurse practitioners has been highlighted as making a difference to patient care (Brykczynski 1989; Fenton 1985). Although both similarities and differences exist among these roles (Fenton and Brykczynski 1993), both roles have been identified as providing high quality nursing care. Evaluation studies have highlighted that the care provided by specialist nurses is clinically effective, efficient and cost effective.

The cost effectiveness of specialist roles has been highlighted in the literature (Kegel 1995; Naylor 1990; Rizzuto 1993). Discharge planning carried out by Clinical Nurse Specialists has been found to reduce the length of stay for patients in hospitals as well as reducing re-admission rates (Chuk 1997; Kegel 1995; Naylor 1990). A randomised controlled trial of 60 asthma patients identified that the information provided to patients by CNSs was found to improve the patient's inhaler technique and understanding of asthma in comparison to information provided at an asthma centre by a general nurse (Donaghy 1995). A meta-analysis of Nurse Practitioners information giving has emphasized that the care and information provided to patients in the primary care sector was no different to care carried out by doctors (Brown and Grimes 1995). Wilson-Barnett and Beech's (1994) meta-analysis evaluated the outcomes of nurse specialists and supported existing research that emphasized nurse specialists provide high quality nursing care that is cost effective.

Other studies have focused on identifying the characteristics that are attributed to expert care. Benner's pioneering work among expert nurses (Benner 1984; Benner and Tanner 1987) drew upon the work of Dreyfus and Dreyfus (1986) in the early sixties. Skill acquisition and the progression from novice to expert were used to emphasise that the quality of patient care was enhanced when provided by expert nurses. Other studies support Benner's (1984) findings (Brykczynski 1989; Chuk 1997; Fenton and Brykczynski 1993). These studies have also explored the characteristics associated with expert nursing care and identified competencies that demonstrate expertise in nursing practice (Brykczynski 1989; Fenton 1985). Their hermeneutic research involved both observations of clinical nurse specialists and nurse practitioners in the clinical environment, which was followed up with interviews among expert nurses across a variety of specialist areas in America.

An evaluation report on promoting action on clinical effectiveness (Dopson *et al.* 1999) identified over a two-year period (PACE 1995–98) that various attributing factors were related to enhancing clinical effectiveness within hospitals. From their sixteen project sites across England, they highlighted the following contributing factors for promoting clinical effectiveness: organisational integration; the influence of key opinion leaders; and the strength and importance of the evidence available. It is noteworthy that their findings identified that 'evidence was found to be more powerful when it chimed with experiential knowledge' (Dopson *et al.* 1999, p. 6). This has implications for clinical practice where the theory and practice gap are drawn closer together, recognising that experience and evidence go hand in hand. Therefore highly skilled and experienced nurses are probably the most suitable people to evaluate current evidence in light of their experience. Relationships between expert opinion and evidence were also found to influence the credibility of the research (Dopson *et al.* 1999).

The multifaceted roles that are most commonly associated with the role of the CNS are the role of the educator, researcher, consultant, expert practitioner and change agent (Hamric and Spross 1989; Miller 1995; Schneider 1992; Vitello-Cicciu 1984). Other roles that have been highlighted include the role of the CNS as an entrepreneur and collaborator (Hazeleton 1993) and a person who takes care of their colleagues (Schaefer 1991). A Delphi study of expert nurses identified 13 characteristics that were found to be prevalent among expert practitioners in nursing, health visiting and midwifery (Butterworth and Bishop 1995). Their findings highlighted that the quality of patient care was improved. This related to individuals involvement in standard setting and also emphasised how the expert practitioners provided a supportive learning environment for their colleague's professional development.

The most common fields of care for CNS exist in diabetes, palliative care and continence nursing (McGee *et al.* 1996). Advanced Nurse Practitioner roles however span the secondary and primary healthcare sectors (Cox 2000a). The multifaceted roles of the CNS/NP place them in an ideal position to develop clinically effective care in the current climate of nursing in which evidence based care takes centre stage.

Research Design

The design for the project embraced the utilisation of multi-method technique. It involved observations of all CNSs/NPs practice. Subjects were observed in their clinical environment over two to five, eight-hour shifts. During this period of observation and through to August 1999, informal discussions and focus group meetings also took place. Thematic analysis (Hammersley and Atkinson 1983; Polit and Hungler 1991) of the findings exposed key constructs and supporting themes that foster and hinder the ability of the CNSs and NPs to engage in clinically effective care.

Observation of Practice

Observation was carried out from mid January 1999 through to June 1999. During this period of observation, one to one informal discussions were held and regular focus group meetings were conducted from February 1999 through to August 1999. Observation involved understanding the role of the CNSs/NPs, the characteristics and activities of their individual roles and recognition of the rules and routines, which encompassed their role. The areas observed throughout the period of observation reflected aspects of observational research that are highlighted by Whyte (1955) and Bruyn (1966). Extensive field notes were made during the observations.

Sampling

A purposive sample as described by Mackenzie (1994) was approached for this study since a specific type of sample was required in order to carry out the research objectives. Selecting an adequate and relevant sample is essential in qualitative research in order to be able to study and focus on the phenomenon of interest. By choosing individuals who are knowledgeable and experienced in the area being studied, the aims of the study can be addressed (Burgess 1982; Morse 1991).

In England there is no universal definition for the CNS and NP role. There are also no universal standards for the educational preparation of CNSs or NPs. This, according to the specialists and nurse practitioners participating in this study is an area that requires clarification. Criteria for inclusion in the study were that the CNSs and NPs were practicing within the Trust.

Recruitment of Subjects to the Study

Access to the Trust was obtained through the Director of Nursing following local ethics committee approval to undertake the research. An introductory meeting to explain the research project was held in October 1998 by the principal investigator. CNSs and NPs working in the Trust were invited to the meeting to discuss the aim and objectives of the research and the rationale for undertaking the research. Following on from this meeting, all CNSs/NPs in the Trust were invited to participate in the research. Fourteen CNSs/NPs were initially recruited from the following specialties across the Trust:

- Oncology/Palliative care
- Cardiology
- Respiratory
- Obstetrics
- Vascular
- Gastroenterology
- Endocrinology

By April data from six CNSs/NPs had to be withdrawn from the study because the nurses commenced employment in other Trusts. A further six nurses were recruited from the following specialties:

- Accident and Emergency
- Intensive therapy
- Rheumatology

A total of twenty CNSs/NPs were observed in their clinical environment over a five-month period. These nurses also engaged in the informal discussions and focus group meetings.

Biographical Data

Biographical information was obtained from all CNSs/NPs that participated in the study by postal questionnaire. Information included qualifications, years worked, areas of work, educational experience, gender, age and grade. The Grades of the CNSs/NPs ranged from F to I. Forty-five per cent of the CNSs/NPs were Grade H. In terms of years of work experience, 35 per cent had been practicing as either a CNS or NP from between one to three years.

Half of the participants in the study had a Bachelor of Science degree; none had Masters degrees. Twenty per cent held diplomas and 55 per cent had more than two English National Board qualifications recorded on the United Kingdom Central Council for Nurses, Midwives and Health Visitors Register. At the time of the study, 45 per cent of the CNSs/NPs were engaged in part-time study, 20 per cent were on BSc. pathways, 15 per cent were studying for a Masters degree and a further ten per cent were engaged in studying English National Board approved specialist courses.

Focus Group Meetings

There were six focus group meetings held between February and August 1999. The principal investigator, research assistant and a few of the CNSs/NPs attended these meetings. There was generally poor attendance at the meetings among the CNSs/NPs due to clinical obligations; attendance by these nurses was generally 30 per cent. The focus group meetings centred on discussing the themes that were emerging from the data analysis. Each meeting was tape-recorded; recordings were transcribed and analysed. Findings from the observations, informal discussions during observations and the focus group meetings were used to develop the key constructs and supporting themes that are presented in this chapter. These also formed the basis for the questionnaire that was circulated nationally. Focus group meetings formed an integral aspect of the research process and were an essential tool to monitor the quality of the research. The CNSs/NPs actively contributed to the discussions associated with observations of their practice.

Construction of Field Notes

A pocket notebook was carried at all times during the observations of the CNSs/NPs practice. Notes were written throughout the duration of each shift. Observations in the clinical environment and dialogue among the researcher and practitioners, their colleagues and patients were documented in the notebook. Care was taken to avoid taking notes during patient contact in order to refrain from distracting the practitioners from their work. During non-observational phases, the notes were read and additional information, which was written in note form, was clarified. The notebook remained with the researcher at all times.

Data Analysis

The field notes from the observations were transcribed, the transcripts were read repeatedly in order to become more familiar with the data and identify key (themes) constructs and supporting categories that were beginning to emerge from the data (Hammersley and Atkinson 1990, 1983; Polit and Hungler 1991). Thematic analysis by writing notes in the margin of the transcripts (Miles and Huberman 1994) identified common themes that were being brought to light from the data (See Table 2.1). Dual code formation (Hinds *et al.* 1989) was approached to ensure the reliability and validity of the data interpretation (Lincoln and Guba 1985; Silverman 1993). In this project, issues of conformability and credibility, which equate to reliability and validity (Lincoln and Guba 1985) in relation to the findings, were substantiated by the CNSs/NPs during the focus group meetings.

Qualitative Research

The richness of understanding an individual's subjective perceptions and experiences is the essence of qualitative research. Its roots are embedded in the philosophy of a naturalistic approach to inquiry that is exploratory in nature. Qualitative research has often been described as being a method of inquiry from the inside by drawing on an individual's life experiences. Miles and Huberman (1994) indicate that qualitative research is a mode of systematic inquiry concerned with understanding human beings and the nature of their transactions both with themselves and their surroundings.

The essence of understanding peoples' behaviour and attitudes to various concepts is rooted in the epistemology of pragmatism, phenomenology,

Table 2.1 Key Constructs and Supporting Themes Identified through Thematic Analysis

Smoothing the way forward	*Disorganisation*
1. Negotiation of clinical decisions	1. Role fragmentation
2. Educating and guiding junior colleagues	2. Role confusion

ethnography and naturalism. The richness in description, and vivid and detailed portrayals of experience, concentrates on the subjectivity and individuality of the subjects being researched. Matza (cited in Hammersley and Atkinson 1983) has indicated that naturalism is a philosophical view that remains true to the nature of the phenomenon under study. This statement emphasises the importance of studying and observing the phenomenon in the context in which it exists.

Four areas identified by Lincoln and Guba (1985) address rigour in qualitative research. These are auditability, conformability, credibility and transferability (Lincoln and Guba 1985). By providing a decision trail, that is a description of how the study was undertaken, the reader can understand how the research was conducted and how the findings were interpreted through exemplars. Koch (1996) emphasises that by precisely stating how the study was conducted and confirming how the data was interpreted it is thereby recognized as encompassing rigour.

Credibility of research findings addresses the issue of how accurately the findings are represented (Erlandson *et al.* 1993). The subjective and interpretative nature of qualitative research questions, whether the findings are drawn from an understanding of the phenomenon being studied or whether the interpretation is a result of the researcher's bias. Therefore, the interpretation of findings must be confirmed by an expert panel review. Hypothesis generation and testing, as has been undertaken in the study, also substantiates credibility.

Koch (1996 p. 192) indicates, 'all meaning requires interpretation'. However all understanding is open to interpretation because we all have different experiences and understanding. It is the concern of qualitative research to provide truthful and believable findings so that readers can be confident that the findings are actually due to the focus of inquiry and not due to the bias of the researcher (Sandelowski 1986; Erlandson *et al.* 1993). Therefore, as indicated above, a review and confirmation of the accuracy of the interpretation of the findings by experts enhances the trustworthiness of the interpretation.

Qualitative research is context bound, since every research situation is about a particular subject in a particular context (Sandelowski 1986). However the richness and beauty of qualitative research generates 'thick description' (Erlandson *et al.* 1993, pp. 31–3; Lincoln and Guba 1985, p. 327) about a phenomenon that can be understood by other people in different contexts so that they can make tentative judgments about the applicability of research findings to their contexts.

Research Findings

Findings from the observations of practice, informal discussions and the focus group meetings are presented in two parts: part one reflects areas that enhance clinical effectiveness and part two reflects areas that act as barriers and hinder the development of clinically effective care.

Enhancing Clinical Effectiveness: Smoothing the Way Forward

Smoothing the way forward is a central theme in enhancing clinical effectiveness. This describes how the CNSs/NPs manage everyday problems, which may or may not be related to their clinical field. The CNSs/NPs use their high level of expertise and knowledge to identify both actual and potential clinical problems relating to patient care. They negotiate clinical decisions with members of the multidisciplinary team, educate their junior colleagues to employ mechanisms that enhance clinically effective care and guide nurses through the daily conundrum of patient care.

It became apparent through data analysis that *smoothing the way forward* is a theme that acts as an umbrella for the following areas:

1. negotiating clinical decisions with members of the multidisciplinary team (MDT);
2. educating and guiding junior colleagues.

Negotiating Clinical Decisions with Members of the MDT

Negotiation is an integral aspect of the CNSs/NPs role. Their expertise and knowledge in their field of specialty place them in an ideal position to identify, prioritise and rationalise problems relating to the nursing care of their patients. The majority of the CNSs/NPs recognise that nursing staff rely on them to negotiate patient problems. One NP stated:

> They often do this to me, call me and get me to sort out stuff with the doctors, rather than do it themselves.

The CNSs/NPs are regularly approached by the ward staff to intervene with the medical staff on issues relating to a patient's treatment. When this issue was discussed during the focus group meetings the CNSs/NPs acknowledged that their experience and knowledge enable them to rationalise their interventions. They also indicated that their junior colleagues trust their judgment and recognize that as CNSs/NPs they have more autonomy and a status which provides them with more power to negotiate patient problems. This is highlighted by the following exemplar:

> I suppose it is because we get the message across much more clearer and that we are also aware of the up to date research being done in a particular area. We are also more likely to be listened to.

Educating and Guiding Junior Colleagues

A high level of rapport between the CNSs/NPs and their colleagues was observed in the clinical environment. The CNSs/NPs are involved in supporting and educating junior nurses and medical staff. They are considered to be a *fountain of knowledge* by most of the junior doctors and are readily approached for advice relating to patient care. One CNS described himself as:

> A walking, talking resource centre.

The CNSs/NPs maintain an important and interactive role in teaching their junior colleagues. The CNSs/NPs actively encourage their junior nurses to recognize the importance of evaluating their nursing interventions in light of the current evidence. Their enthusiasm for sharing their knowledge is evident when they are approached for advice. As facilitators the CNSs/NPs actively support the professional development of their junior colleagues and encourage individuals to provide evidence based care by discussing and critically appraising current research in their particular field.

It was noted during the observation phase of the project, that the Cardiac CNS would usually be approached by other nurses and junior doctors to clarify a particular ECG interpretation, or to discuss anxieties a junior nurse or doctor might have in regards to a particular patient responding to a given treatment. It was found that the CNS/NP is usually the *first port of call.* Professional recognition by fellow nurses reinforces the role of the CNS/NP in educating and guiding junior colleagues. However the medical staff rarely demonstrated such enthusiasm in relation to professional recognition.

On occasions the CNS/NP is even approached to discuss personal problems staff have. The CNSs/NPs actively provide support and guidance to nursing colleagues. In the focus group meetings, a number of the CNSs/NPs would jovially announce that they often felt as though they were perceived as a social worker, a counsellor and a trouble shooter, all wrapped into one neat package.

In conclusion, negotiation, education and guidance smooth the way forward. However, there are certain issues that act as a barrier and hinder clinically effective care.

Barriers to Clinical Effectiveness: Disorganisation

Disorganisation is the central theme in creating barriers to clinical effectiveness. Disorganisation is evidenced through:

1. role fragmentation;
2. role confusion.

Role Fragmentation

The CNSs/NPs are approached by junior nurses to *unload* their daily problems relating to the clinical environment (for example, staff shortages or poor skill mix). Over the five months of observation, it became common practice to observe the CNSs/NPs being called upon to cover staff shortages during breaks, cover a full shift on the wards or to *chip in* on the clinical units/ wards to administer intravenous medications.

For example, on one occasion, a CNS received a telephone call just as observation was to be concluded for the day, from one of the medical wards. Four patients had not received their intravenous antibiotics because of a poor skill mix and staff shortages on the ward. Although the CNS *chipped in* because she felt obliged to ensure that adequate nursing care was being delivered to the patients, the CNS indicated this hindered her from focusing on her role.

The following exemplar, highlights how an Emergency Nurse Practitioner is prevented from utilising her specialist skills and expertise:

> I love being an ENP. We follow the patient through from admission through to discharge, they don't see anybody else which makes their whole experience less traumatic. I make a thorough assessment of their condition and a diagnosis then give them health advice and send them on their way. You can't get more holistic care than that. However, I hardly get a chance to be an ENP because of staff shortages. In fact, today I am being an ENP in honour of your arrival [Subject laughs], because that is what you wanted to see me do!

Noticeably, *chipping in* is only a temporary measure and not a permanent solution to staff shortages. Consequently the CNSs/NPs are not utilising their expertise and knowledge thoroughly. By *chipping in* they are drawn further and further away from their specialist role. The CNSs/NPs appear to spend a considerable amount of time *sorting out a lot of mess* before they can actually perform the role they should be undertaking.

The following exemplar highlights frustration experienced by a CNS.

> I spend half my time doing all these errands because there is nobody employed to do these jobs. I feel like a Jack-of-all- trades and master of none. I am supposed to be a clinical nurse specialist but rarely get the opportunity to do what I am supposed to be doing. That patient needs me to sit with her and discuss how she is coping with the Chemo, not have me disappear every half an hour to run and get the next patient's notes.

Role fragmentation is a category where data reflects that the majority of nurses find it an *uphill struggle* to deliver the high quality nursing care which they want to deliver. They often feel that they are 'drawn into jobs which should be done by others', and consequently feel that they are doing the jobs of many people while they attempt to make ends meet.

Role Confusion

Role fragmentation creates role confusion among some of the CNSs/NPs and, indeed, their colleagues. Role fragmentation caused by *chipping in* when there are staff shortages, for example, has lead to CNSs/NPs modifying their role on a daily basis. In order to resolve this issue, CNSs/NPs indicate that role clarification must be addressed by the Trust.

Some staff do not appear to recognize that by drawing the CNSs/NPs into problems related to staffing shortages, for example, they are prohibiting the CNS/NP from maximising their full potential as specialist nurses and practitioners. By relying on the CNSs/NPs, staff demonstrate they do not seem to understand the role of the CNS/NP. For example, while observing a Diabetic CNS practice, a doctor bleeped the CNS to ask if the CNS could confirm the sliding scale dosage for a patient. After discussing the dosage the doctor asked the CNS to come up to the ward and start the sliding scale because the doctor was busy. The CNS explained that she was in the middle of assessing patients in the clinic and would not be able to come up to the ward. After putting the phone down, the CNSs turned and said:

> It feels good to know that doctors ask our advice, however they still don't see us as specialists. That doctor saw me filling in on the wards the other evening and probably thinks that although I know my stuff really well, I am really here as a spare hand. That's the problem, they don't understand how nurses can be specialists!

Role confusion was most noticeable among CNSs/NPs in new positions. They appeared to *struggle* to clarify their responsibilities and expectations. Some new CNSs/NPs indicated they 'feel as though everybody is taking a chunk out of me'. They feel confused about what their role entails. In these instances it was identified through the observations and in the focus groups that 'a lack of clinical supervision and peer guidance' was also responsible for some aspects of role confusion.

Conclusion and Recommendations for Enhancing Practice

The findings from this exploratory study indicate that the expertise and knowledge of the CNSs/NPs place them in an ideal position to develop and promote clinically effective care. However barriers identified through the research impede the role of the CNSs/NPs and subsequently have a negative impact on clinical effectiveness. The following recommendations are made for enhancing clinical effectiveness.

1. Undertaking a comprehensive review of all job descriptions of the CNSs and NPs. This should be undertaken collaboratively with the CNSs and NPs aimed at achieving a consensus of agreement regarding main duties and key tasks.
2. Elimination of barriers to clinically effective care so that aspects of advanced practice, such as physical assessment skills and diagnosis, can be assumed. This could be achieved if role clarification occurred.
3. Provision of clinical supervision to all CNSs/NPs, which is essential to the development of the individual CNSs/NPs practice. Clinical supervision should take place regularly as this has been shown to enhance clinical practice and is especially so in demanding roles (Watson 1999). New CNSs/NPs would particularly benefit from regular supervision and contact with other CNSs/NPs from their specialties. Through this activity the CNSs/NPs will learn from each other by sharing their experiences and ways in which they have resolved difficult situations.
4. Regular audits and evaluations of practice should occur, as these will enable role clarification by acknowledging the interventions carried out by the CNSs/NPs. Regular audits and evaluations of practice will identify areas of practice that need to be improved as well as provide an avenue for recognizing clinically effective care. The research found that not all CNSs/NPs are involved in the audit process that has been developed in the Trust. The involvement of all CNSs/NPs in audit should be initiated through a Clinical Governance/Shared Governance Model of Nursing (Cox 2000b).
5. Study for the Clinical Nurse Specialists and Nurse Practitioners should be encouraged at Masters level. Clinical Nurse Specialists and Nurse Practitioners should be allocated study time in order to undertake further education. In-house training should also be offered as a mechanism for developing clinical skills. It is recommended programmes which feature clinical skills development, such as physical assessment, be offered as part of the in-house training clinical specialists and nurse practitioners receive.

References

Benner, P. (1984) *From Novice to Expert: Excellence and Power in Clinical Nursing Practice*, California, Addison Wesley

Benner, P. and C. Tanner (1987) 'Clinical Judgment: How Expert Nurses use Intuition', *American Journal of Nursing*, 87(1) pp. 23–31

Brown, S. and D. Grimes (1995) 'A Meta-analysis of Nurse Practitioners and Nurse Midwives in Primary Care', *Nursing Research*, 44(6) pp. 332–9

Brykczynski, K. (1989) 'An Interpretive Study Describing the Clinical Judgement of Nurse Practitioners', *Scholarly Inquiry for Nursing Practice: An International Journal*, 3(2) pp. 75–104

Burgess, R. (1982) *Field Research: a sourcebook and field manual*, London George Allen and Unwin

Butterworth, T. and V. Bishop (1995) 'Identifying the Characteristics of Optimum Practice: findings from a survey of practice experts in nursing, midwifery and health visiting', *Journal of Advanced Nursing*, 22(1) pp. 24–32

Bruyn, S. (1966) *The Human Perspective in Sociology: the methodology of participant observation*, New Jersey, Prentice-Hall

Chuk, P. (1997) 'Clinical Nurse Specialists and Quality Patient Care', *Journal of Advanced Nursing*, 26(3) pp. 501–6

Cox, C. (2000a) 'The Nurse Consultant: An Advanced Nurse Practitioner?' *Nursing Times*, 96(13) p. 48

Cox, Carol L. (2000b) 'Clinical Governance and Shared Governance', *Practice Nursing*, 11(16) pp. 17–20

Department of Health (1997) *The New NHS Modern and Dependable*, London, HMSO

Department of Health (1998) *A First class Service: Quality in the New NHS*, London, HMSO

Department of Health (1999a) *Clinical Governance: Quality in the New NHS*, Leeds, NHSE

Department of Health (1999b) *National Institute for Clinical Excellence*, London, HMSO

Donaghy, D. (1995) 'The Asthma Specialist and Patient Education', *Professional Nurse*, 11(3) pp. 160–2

Dopson, S., J. Gabbay, J. Locock and D. Chambers (1999) *Evaluation of the PACE Programme: final report*, Oxford Health Care Management Institute, Tempelton College, University of Oxford, Wessex Institute for Health Research and Development, University of Southampton

Dreyfus, H. and S. Dreyfus (1986) *Mind Over Machine; the power of human intuition and expertise in the era of the computer*, New York, Free Press

Erlandson, D., E. Harris, B. Skipper and S. Allen (1993) *Doing Naturalistic Inquiry: a Guide to Methods*, California, Sage

Fenton, M. (1985) 'Identifying Competencies of Clinical Nurse Specialists', *Journal of Nursing Administration*, 15(12) pp. 16–20

Fenton, M. and Brykczynski, K. (1993) 'Qualitative Distinctions and Similarities in the Practice of Clinical Nurse Specialists and Nurse Practitioners', *Journal of Professional Nursing*, 9(6) pp. 313–26

Hammersley, M. and P. Atkinson (1983) *Ethnography: Principals in Practice*, London, Tavistock

Hammersley, M. and P. Atkinson (1990) *Reading Ethnographic Research: A Critical Guide*, London, Longman

Hamric, A. and J. Spross (1989) *The Clinical Nurse Specialist in Theory and Practice*, Philadelphia, W.B. Saunders

Hazeleton, J. (1993) 'Clinical Nurse Specialist Sub Roles: foundations for entrepreneurship', *Clinical Nurse Specialist*, 7(1) pp. 40–5

Hicks, C. (1997) 'Research: the dilemma of incorporating research into clinical practice', *British Journal of Nursing*, 6(9) pp. 511–15

Hinds, P., S. Scandrett-Hibden and L. McCauley (1989) 'Further Assessment of a Method to Estimate Reliability and Validity of Qualitative Research Findings', *Journal of Advanced Nursing*, 15(4) pp. 235–41

Kegel, L. (1995) 'Advanced Practice Nurses Can Refine the Management of Heart Failure', *Clinical Nurse Specialist* 9(2) pp. 76–81

Koch, T. (1996) 'Implementation of a Hermeneutic Inquiry in Nursing: Philosophy, Rigor and Representation', *Journal of Advanced Nursing*, 24(1) pp. 174–84

Lincoln, Y. and E. Guba (1985) *Naturalistic Enquiry*, California, Sage.

Mackenzie, A. (1994) 'Evaluating Ethnography: Considerations for Analysis', *Journal of Advanced Nursing*, 19(4) pp. 774–81

McGee, P., G. Casteldine and R. Brown (1996) 'A Survey of Specialist and Advanced Nursing Practice in England', *British Journal of Nursing*, 5(11) pp. 683–6

Miller, S. (1995) 'The Clinical Nurse Specialist: a way forward?' *Journal of Advanced Nursing*, 22(3) pp. 494–501

Miles, M. and A. Huberman (1994) *An Expanded Source Book: Qualitative Data Analysis*, London, Sage

Morse, J. (1991) *Qualitative Nursing Research: A Contemporary Dialogue*, London, Sage

National Health Service Executive (1996) *Achieving Effective Practice: A clinical effectiveness and research information pack for nurses, midwives and health visitors*, Leeds, NHSE

Naylor, M. (1990) 'Comprehensive Discharge Planning for Hospitalised Elderly: a pilot study', *Nurse Researcher*, 39(3) pp. 156–61

Polit, D. and B. Hungler (1991) *Nursing Research, Principles and Methods*, 4th edn, London, J.B. Lippincott

Rizzuto, C. (1993) 'Issues in Clinical Nursing Research: documenting clinical nurse specialist role functions and outcomes', *Western Journal of Nursing Research*, 17(4) pp. 448–50

Royal College of Nursing (1996) *Clinical Effectiveness, A Royal College of Nursing Guide*, London, Royal College of Nursing

Sandelowski, M. (1986) 'The Problem of Rigor in Qualitative Research', *Advances in Nursing Science*, 3(3) pp. 27–37

Schaefer, K. (1991) 'Taking Care of the Caretakers: a partial explanation of clinical nurse specialist practice', *Journal of Advanced Nursing*, 16(3) pp. 270–6

Schneider, J. (1992) 'Clinical Nurse Specialist: role definition as discharge planning coordinator', *Clinical Nurse Specialist*, 6(1) pp. 36–9

Silverman, D. (1993) *Interpreting Qualitative Data*, Gower, Hants, Aldershot

Vitello-Cicciu, J. (1984) 'Excellence in Critical Care: educating the clinical specialists', *Critical Care Quarterly*, 7(1) pp. 26–32

Watson, J. (1999) *Postmodern Nursing and Beyond*, Edinburgh, Churchill Livingstone

Wilson-Barnett, J. and Beech, S. (1994) 'Evaluating the Clinical Nurse Specialists: A Review', *International Journal of Nursing Studies*, 31(6) pp. 561–71

Whyte, W. (1955) *Street Corner Society*, Chicago, University of Chicago Press.

CHAPTER 3

Clinical Effectiveness and the Realities of Practice: a National Quantitative Study

CAROL LYNN COX AND SONYA AHLUWALIA

Introduction

This chapter follows on from Chapter 2 and describes the findings of a quantitative pilot study that aimed to discern whether the findings from the qualitative study could be substantiated nationally amongst a convenience sample of Clinical Nurse Specialists (CNSs) and Nurse Practitioners (NPs) who work in the National Health Service (NHS) and private healthcare facilities. With the introduction of the government's initiatives aimed at modernising the National Health Service (DoH 1997; 1998a., 1998b) it is postulated among many CNSs/NPs that the complexities of delivering care to patients have increased. These specialist nurses indicate that, due to these complexities, they are experiencing increased stressors in relation to their work. The research project described in this chapter was an extension of the study described in Chapter 2. This project like the qualitative study was funded by the Central and East London Education Consortium (CELEC). It commenced in December 1999 and was completed in June 2000. The study has confirmed areas that foster and hinder the practice of the CNS and NP in relation to the provision of clinically effective care and has identified areas that are significantly impacting on the ability of these specialist nurses to deliver what they perceive to be high quality, cost effective care. In light of the findings, recommendations for practice enhancement are explicated in the conclusion of this chapter.

To place the present chapter in context a brief review of the qualitative study is described and then the findings from the quantitative pilot study are presented. In relation to the qualitative study, multi-method technique was used to discern how clinically effective care is fostered and hindered among CNSs and NPs. Qualitative approaches included non-participant observation of practice, interviews during observation and focus group discussions and meetings. The quantitative approach involved the construction and pilot testing of a questionnaire that validated qualitative findings through non-parametric statistical analysis. Areas found to foster clinically effective care in the qualitative research project were related to *Smoothing the Way Forward*. These are:

1. negotiating clinical decisions with members of the multi-disciplinary team (MDT);
2. educating and guiding junior colleagues.

Areas found to hinder the ability of the CNS and NP to engage in or provide clinically effective nursing care are related to *Disorganisation*. These are:

1. role fragmentation;
2. role confusion.

Of major significance in the quantitative pilot study, is the correlation of findings from the qualitative research in Newham Healthcare NHS Trust with the experiences of CNSs and NPs working in other NHS trusts and private healthcare facilities throughout England. Correlation indicates there is no significant difference ($p > 0.05$) between practice experience of specialist nurses at the test Trust and other NHS Trusts and private healthcare facilities throughout England. Factors that foster and hinder the ability of the CNSs and NPs to engage in and provide clinically effective nursing care are the same throughout England.

The pilot study has confirmed the reliability and validity of the questionnaire. It has also confirmed that the expertise and knowledge of CNSs and NPs places them in an ideal position to develop and promote clinically effective care. However the barriers identified through the quantitative research impede the role of the CNS and NP and subsequently have a negative impact on clinical effectiveness.

Research Questions and Aims of the Study

The questions that drove the study were 'are the areas that foster and hinder clinically effective care amongst Clinical Nurse Specialists and Nurse Practitioners at the test Trust the same as those experienced amongst Clinical Nurse Specialists and Nurse Practitioners Nationally?' If the answer to question one is yes, then 'what are the most significant and insignificant areas that foster and hinder the provision of clinically effective care amongst Clinical Nurse Specialists and Nurse Practitioners Nationally?'

The aims of the research were to identify whether there were significant similarities or differences between the responses among the two groups of CNSs and NPs and to identify the most significant areas that foster and hinder the provision of clinically effective care among CNSs and NPs nationally.

Review of the Literature and Rationale for the Study

Providing evidenced based nursing care by Advanced Nurse Practitioners to patients has been shown to be efficient, cost effective and a fundamental component of clinically effective care (Cox 2000a). It has also been highlighted through research that if practice is evidence based it is more likely to be cost effective, appropriate and justifiable (Cox and Ahluwalia 2000; Hicks 1997). According to the Department of Health, clinical governance is a key component in the provision of evidence based, clinically effective care (DoH 1999a).

Clinical governance has as its underlying premise a duty to care and to continuously improve the quality of services patients receive (Cox 2000b). CNSs and NPs have a duty to provide high standards of care. They can do this by creating an environment in which excellence in clinical care can flourish (Department of Health 1999a; 1999b). Literature indicates clinical governance has important consequences for patient care (for example, best practice) (Castledine 2000a; Wilson and Tingle 1999.) It, therefore, becomes apparent that clinical governance can have a strong influence on the implementation of clinically effective care. However, as stated in Chapter 2, little research has been undertaken in the area of developing clinical effectiveness and clinical governance is in the early stages of development in many healthcare facilities in Britain. According to Castledine (2000a) nurses are rarely viewed as risk takers or leaders in healthcare.

> Institutional policies seem insistent on keeping nurses as managed resources and in multidisciplinary teams where they are unable to assert their authority and lead their medical colleagues towards true inter-professional involvement and shared decision making (Castledine 2000a:670).

Shared decision making is a fundamental part of clinical governance (Cox 2000b). If Castledine's (2000a) statement is correct, it has significant implications for clinical governance and the implementation of clinically effective care. In addition, according to (Dopson *et al.* 1999) few studies have been undertaken that specifically identify how clinical effectiveness is applied to directly influence practice. Therefore, the study described in this chapter has relevance in terms of general perspectives regarding factors that foster and hinder the provision of clinically effective care by CNSs and NPs within the developing clinical governance arena.

For the purpose of this study, the National Health Service Executive (1996) definition of clinical effectiveness quoted in Chapter 1 has been adopted as the working definition:

> Clinical Effectiveness is demonstrated when specific clinical interventions do what they are intended to do, which is to maintain and improve health whilst

securing the greatest possible health gain from available resources. (NHSE 1996, p. 2)

Research Design

The research design for the project described in this chapter was correlational and based on the findings from the qualitative study. To review, the field notes from observations of practice, individual discussions during observation and notes from the focus groups were transcribed. The transcripts were read repeatedly in order to become more familiar with the data and to identify key themes and categories that were beginning to emerge from the data (Hammersley and Atkinson 1983, 1990; Polit and Hungler 1991). Thematic analysis occurred by writing notes in the margin of the transcripts (Miles and Huberman 1994). These notes reflected common threads that were emerging from the data. Dual code formation (Hinds *et al.* 1989) was approached to ensure the reliability and validity of the data interpretation (Lincoln and Guba 1985; Silverman 1993). These findings were then discussed in the focus group meetings. These discussions substantiated the credibility and consistency (Lincoln and Guba 1985) of the themes that were emerging. The key constructs and supporting themes that were identified during this process were transformed into empirical indicators (situations that foster and hinder the provision of clinically effective care). These were used to develop the questionnaire.

Correlational design is used when the investigators suspect a relationship exists among variables and can support their suspicions through literature or previous research (Brink and Wood 1998). The variables are known to exist in the population being studied and possible connections can be made among the variables. The purpose of a correlational study is to determine the relationship among the variables. Correlational designs are beyond the level of descriptive designs in that the investigator does not examine variables at random, but looks at specific variables and scrutinises the relationship among the variables.

Questionnaire Development

A panel of experts was recruited to discuss findings, which arose from thematic analysis and to agree the empirical indicators that would be tested on the questionnaire. Percentage of agreement at 80 per cent or greater was used as the standard in determining whether an empirical indicator would be listed on the questionnaire. As previously indicated, content of the questionnaire (see Appendix Table A 3.1) was based on the key constructs and supporting themes identified from the non-participant observations, informal discussions and the focus group meetings. The key constructs and supporting themes were:

- Role confusion;
- Negotiation;
- Role fragmentation;
- Educator;
- Professional recognition;
- CNS/NP as a counsellor;
- Role development.

The panel of experts was established by contacting CNSs/NPs from the Royal London Hospitals' NHS Trust, City and Hackney NHS Trust, Homerton Hospital NHS Trust and Newham Community NHS Trust. Twenty-eight CNSs/NPs were recruited and provided with background information about the study and asked to undertake a content analysis of the questionnaire. CNSs/NPs who were able to attend the introductory meeting were provided with an overview of the project and a copy of the questionnaire. CNSs and NPs unable to attend the meeting were posted a copy of the questionnaire and asked to examine the contents and to comment on the statements on the questionnaire.

Consensus on the content – through percentage of agreement – of the questionnaire was reached after two rounds of content analysis. This process took six weeks to complete. A percentage of agreement of 83 per cent was achieved in round one (N=38 out of 46 statements), and round two had a percentage of agreement of 92 per cent (N=35 out of the 38 statements). This gives the questionnaire a confidence interval of .9. The information provided in a confidence interval of .9 is of considerable interest. It provides a strategy for hypothesis testing that defines all possible null hypotheses (empirical indicators). In practice, a confidence interval of .7 or above is highly significant. A researcher need never test null hypotheses in this situation. Null hypothesis testing can be bypassed and all research questions can be answered directly in terms of the confidence interval (McLaughlin and Marascuilo 1990).

Content validity and construct validity were determined by the panel of experts confirming the content of the questionnaire through percentage of agreement and by pilot testing the questionnaire. The questionnaire was formatted (Table A 3.3) and piloted in December 1999, amongst a convenience sample (N=35) of CNSs/NPs from NHS Trusts and other healthcare facilities throughout England who were employed in the public and private sector.

Biographical Data Questionnaire

The same questionnaire (Table A 3.2) that was used to collect biographical information in the qualitative study was sent to all CNSs/NPs that participated in the study. The qualifications, work and educational experience of all the CNSs/NPs participating in the study were recorded.

Subjects

A purposive convenience sample (Mackenzie 1994) of CNSs and NPs was obtained for this study since a particular sample was required in order to address the research aims. Selecting an adequate and relevant sample is essential in order to be able to study and focus on the phenomenon of interest, therefore, by choosing individuals who are knowledgeable and experienced in these areas, the aims of the study can be addressed (Burgess 1982; Morse 1991).

Access to the nurse specialists was through direct contact via City University where they were studying for a Masters degree. Permission for access to the nurse specialists was gained from the Dean of the School of Nursing and Midwifery and the Course Director for the Masters degree programme. Information about the study was provided and agreement to participate in the study was determined by the subjects responding to the questions on the questionnaire and returning the questionnaire to the Course Director of the Masters degree programme. All questionnaires were responded to anonymously.

Specialist practice among the sample included oncology, palliative care, critical care, accident and emergency, respiratory, infectious diseases, TB, HIV/AIDS, midwifery, tissue viability, vascular, gastroenterology, gerontology, endocrinology, haematology and rheumatology.

Biographical Data

As previously indicated, the qualifications, work and educational experience of all the CNSs/NPs participating in the study were recorded (Table A 3.2). Grades the CNSs/NPs held ranged from F to I; 40 per cent of the CNSs/NPs were Grade H. In terms of years of work experience, 65 per cent had been practicing as either a CNS or NP from between two to five years.

Educationally, only one of the CNSs/NPs had a Masters degree. Sixty-five per cent of the participants in the study had a first degree. Fifteen per cent held diplomas and the remainder held certificates in nursing. As in the qualitative study, 55 per cent had more than two English National Board qualifications recorded on the United Kingdom Central Council for Nurses, Midwives and Health Visitors Register. At the time of the study, due to the nature of the convenience sample, all of the CNSs/NPs were studying for a Masters degree on a part time basis including the nurse with a masters degree from a previous course of study.

Method of Testing and Analysing the Questionnaire

The questionnaire (Table A 3.3) was pilot tested on a convenience sample of (N=35) CNSs and NPs. Responses to the questionnaire were analysed using the statistical software package for the social sciences (SPSS) version 8. Seven independent variables were tested:

1. Role fragmentation;
2. Role confusion;
3. Educating junior colleagues;
4. Negotiation of patient problems;
5. Professional recognition;
6. Role development;
7. Taking care of junior colleagues.

Frequency Distributions

When a substantial number of observations or measurements have been made, it is useful to organise data into classes according to the magnitude of the measurement. Grouping data into classes make interpretation of the results easier. A frequency distribution is a table in which values for a variable are grouped into classes and the number of observed values that belong in each class are recorded. Data organised in a frequency distribution are called grouped data. Frequency tables can be used to check the accuracy and consistency of data. A frequency table is a display of a set of categories with the number or percentage of instances observed in each category listed. These tables can be used to detect data entry and data processing errors. Potential sources of bias can also be detected. The data provided can inform readers to understand and evaluate the outcomes of a survey.

Mann-Whitney U Test

The Mann-Whitney U Test for two independent samples was used to analyse the results of individual responses to empirical indicators delineated on the questionnaire. This statistical test is a non-parametric test. It makes no assumptions about the sample's population distribution. This particular analysis is used to compare the responses among two independent groups of sampled data and draws a parallel to the independent T test used for parametric analysis.

The alternate hypothesis was tested in an attempt to falsify the results found at Newham Healthcare NHS Trust. The alternate hypothesis is: *there are significant differences between the responses amongst the two groups of clinical nurse specialists and nurse practitioners and additionally these responses will be different than the clinical nurse specialists and nurse practitioners responses at Newham Healthcare NHS Trust.* If the alternate cannot be accepted, then the null hypothesis for this test must be accepted. The null hypothesis is: *there are no significant differences between the responses amongst the two groups of clinical nurse specialists and nurse practitioners and additionally these responses will be the same as those of the clinical nurse specialists and nurse practitioners responses at Newham Healthcare NHS Trust.*

Wilcoxon Rank Sum Test

The Wilcoxon rank sum test is used to test the null hypothesis that the values in two populations are not different in level or magnitude where the values for the two samples are collected as paired observations. The Wilcoxon test is a non-parametric equivalent to the Student's t distribution to test the difference between two means based on paired observations. In a comparison of two sample means such samples are often collected as pairs of values and are, therefore, dependent samples rather than independent samples. The dependent samples do not have to contain the same people in each group, rather the individuals can be matched so that for each individual in one sample group there is an individual in the other sample group with similar characteristics. These types of samples are paired observations or matched pairs. The Wilcoxon test considers the magnitude of differences between the matched pairs and is a more powerful test than the sign test.

Questionnaire Results – Statistical Findings

Frequency Distribution

The responses from the sample (N=35) of 22 Clinical Nurse Specialists (N=22) and 13 Nurse Practitioners (N=13) follow. Individual responses were collated using the SPSS package for frequency tables.

Role fragmentation

Fragmentation of the CNSs/NPs role was an area that the respondents had mixed views about (31.4 per cent disagree, agree 48.6 per cent). There were also mixed responses in regards to CNSs/NPs being drawn into areas that were not related to their specialist role (45.7 per cent disagree, 42.9 per cent agree). A lack of resources was identified as an area responsible for creating role fragmentation (71.4 per cent agree, 11.4 per cent strongly agree).

Role confusion

The majority of the CNSs/NPs agreed that new specialist roles created role confusion (60.0 per cent agree, 25.7 per cent strongly agree). However there were mixed views regarding the CNSs and NPs in new roles as creating role confusion through trial and error in their practice (34.3 per cent strongly disagree, 45.7 per cent agree, 14.3 per cent strongly agree). It was interesting to find that there was a strong percentage of disagreement in regard to specialist roles deskilling the general nurse practice skills on the wards (28.6 per cent disagree, 48.6 per cent strongly disagree). This finding is in direct contradiction to Castledine's (2000b) view published in the *British Journal of Nursing*.

Respondents had mixed views about specialist roles only focusing on their expertise (11.4 per cent disagree, 31.4 per cent strongly disagree, 48.6 per cent agree) but strongly disagreed that role boundaries were established by individual CNSs/NPs on a daily basis (20.0 per cent disagree, 57.1 per cent strongly disagree).

Educating junior colleagues

Almost one hundred per cent agreement was found with regard to the CNSs/NPs educational role (48.6 per cent agree, 42.9 per cent strongly agree). Doctors were another group that were educated by specialist nurses (57.1 per cent agree, 31.4 per cent strongly agree). Similarly, it was perceived that both doctors and nurses were heavily supported in the clinical environment by CNSs/NPs (28.6 per cent agree, 65.7 per cent strongly agree). Apart from the educative role of these nurses, research was an area that most respondents felt the CNSs/NPs were actively involved in (68.6 per cent agree, 31.4 per cent disagree). Over half of the respondents disagreed with the statement that the CNSs/NPs did not have the time to engage in research (51.4 per cent disagree, 8.6 per cent strongly disagree). Therefore, education, research and facilitation were perceived as integral components of the CNSs/NPs role.

Negotiation of patient problems

A high percentage of agreement (43.8 per cent agree, 37.5 per cent strongly agree) was related to the belief that the CNSs/NPs ability to prioritise and rationalise patient problems was due to their high level of experience and knowledge. Half of the respondents perceived that the knowledge and experience among CNSs and NPs placed them in an ideal position to act as troubleshooters (57.1 per cent agree, 34.3 per cent strongly agree). This was clearly indicated by the majority of respondents identifying CNSs/NPs as more autonomous and powerful in clinical decision-making (51.4 per cent agree, 25.7 per cent strongly agree).

Professional recognition

The educative role is supported by the responses relating to a strong agreement that both doctors and nurses value the clinical opinion of CNSs/NPs (Dr: 57.1 per cent agree, 14.3 per cent strongly agree; nurse: 71.4 per cent agree, 22.9 per cent strongly agree). This is substantiated by the strong agreement of over half the respondents where the CNSs/NPs are perceived as the first port of call (45.7 per cent agree, 40.0 per cent strongly agree) in relation to patient care issues. Staff development, peer guidance and support were also areas that were considered essential to the development of the CNSs/NPs role (37.1 per cent agree, 60.0 per cent strongly agree).

Role development

Clinical supervision was perceived as being integral to the role development of the CNSs/NPs (60.0 per cent agree, 22.9 per cent strongly agree). Collaboration among other specialist nurses was also an area that the respondents felt strongly about (34.3 per cent agree, 65.7 per cent strongly agree). Audits to evaluate areas of care were a controversial area, over half of the respondents felt that CNSs/NPs were not involved in the audit process (48.6 per cent agree, 25.7 per cent strongly agree). However, evaluating patient outcomes was considered part of the role of the CNSs/NPs (51.4 per cent agree, 25.7 per cent strongly agree).

Taking care of junior colleagues (counsellor)

An additional role of the CNSs/NPs was identified as providing guidance and support to their junior colleagues (65.7 per cent agree, 14.3 per cent strongly agree). Rapport among these groups was also perceived to exist (62.9 per cent agree, 11.4 per cent strongly agree). The multi-faceted role of CNSs/NPs that has been identified in the literature is supported by the respondents acknowledging the role of the educator – counsellor – facilitator and researcher in their responses on the questionnaire.

Mann-Whitney U Test Results

The responses from the sample (N=35) were comprised of 22 Clinical Nurse Specialists (N=22) and 13 Nurse Practitioners (N=13). Individual responses were collated using the SPSS package.

The Mann-Whitney U Test indicated that there were no significant differences in the correlations of findings between the two groups of respondents:

CNSs and NPs. Both groups had similar responses. It is apparent that both CNSs and NPs have similar experiences and noticeably that the experiences of the CNSs and NPs working at Newham Healthcare NHS Trust are not restricted to the Newham Healthcare Trust. Therefore, Newham Healthcare NHS Trust is not unique in its experiences. Statistical analysis substantiates findings from the observations, informal discussions and focus group meetings that were undertaken in the qualitative part of the research. The results highlight common issues that are being experienced by CNSs and NPs throughout England.

Similar responses between the two groups raises a question regarding how much overlap exists between the role of the CNS and NP. The statistical findings substantiate the qualitative findings at Newham Healthcare NHS Trust with regard to the importance of clarifying the role of CNSs and NPs. In relation to the highest and lowest mean ranks the following results are significant for the CNS and NP.

In relation to the CNS, the highest mean rank on the Mann-Whitney U Test was 20.23. This was in response to the statement that the CNS plays an integral role in educating doctors. The second highest mean rank on the Mann-Whitney U Test was 20.09 in response to the statement that ward staff are sometimes deskilled by the CNS. In relation to the lowest mean rank on the Mann-Whitney U Test the rank was 15.76. This was in response to the statement that the CNS needs to educate doctors, nurses and other members of multidisciplinary team about the role of the CNS.

In relation to the NP, the highest mean rank on the Mann-Whitney U Test was 21.46. This was in response to the statement that the NP needs to demonstrate their clinical credibility before they are recognized as competent by other specialist nurses. The second highest mean rank on the Mann-Whitney U Test was 20.35 in response to the statement that the new specialist roles of the NP are often a case of trial and error. In relation to the lowest mean rank on the Mann-Whitney U Test the rank was 14.23. This was in response to the statement that the NP plays an integral role in educating doctors.

In relation to both groups of nurse specialists, the primary areas that were of most importance to them were in relation to peer support and guidance being necessary for staff development (36.19) and developing their role through clinical supervision (36.05)

Wilcoxon Rank Sum Test

The areas that were significant for both groups of nurse specialists was the expressed need for clinical supervision (ranked sum = 394.5) and the need for staff development in order to develop their expertise (ranked sum = 394.5). The key areas that followed on from this were the concern that they focus only on their area of expertise and do not provide holistic care (ranked sum = 388.0) and that they should periodically collaborate with other nurse specialists in their field in order to exchange ideas and improve client care.

P values were not significant ($p > 0.05$) for any of the seven independent variables (empirical indicators) tested on the questionnaire. Therefore, the alternate hypothesis was rejected and the null hypothesis accepted. In conclusion, the pilot study results (p values for all empirical indicators > 0.05) indicate the experiences of Clinical Nurse Specialists and Nurse Practitioners at Newham Healthcare NHS Trust are experienced by Clinical Nurse Specialists and Nurse Practitioners in similar roles throughout England.

Recommendations for Enhancing Practice

The findings from this pilot study indicate, as they did in the qualitative study, that the expertise and knowledge of the CNSs/NPs place them in an ideal position to implement and promote clinically effective care. Barriers identified in this research impede the role of the CNSs/NPs and subsequently have a negative impact on clinical effectiveness. In the narrative that follows some recommendations for practice are made that have been identified as key activities in enhancing clinical effectiveness.

Education, coaching (guiding) and negotiation are skills the CNSs and NPs are confident they possess and feel make a difference in relation to clinical effectiveness. These factors facilitate clinically effective care. Enhancing these skills can be achieved through peer support and guidance in relation to staff development and the introduction of clinical supervision. This study indicates clinical effectiveness can be achieved through the enhancement of these skills. The CNSs and NPs should be encouraged to extend their own knowledge through English National Board specialist courses at degree level and advanced practice courses at Masters level. In relation to continuous professional development, study should be encouraged at Master's level.

In-house training can be an effective mechanism for developing clinical skills. It is recommended continuous professional development programmes that feature clinical skills development, such as physical assessment, are offered as part of the in-house training CNSs and NPs receive. Competencies associated with clinically effective care such as those described in the National Organisations of Nurse Practitioner Faculties (NONPF 1995) (see Table A 3.4) should be used as the basis for any competency based continuing education programme that is established for the CNSs and NPs. These competencies are associated with Advanced Practice and reflect higher levels of practice delineated by the United Kingdom Central Council for Nurses, Midwives and Health Visitors. The identification of core competencies and standards of practice would resolve some issues associated with role confusion. This view is supported by Castledine (2000b).

Providing clinical supervision to all CNSs/NPs is essential for the development of the individual CNSs/NPs practice. Clinical supervision should take place regularly as this has been shown to enhance clinical practice and especially so in demanding roles (Watson 1999). New CNSs/NPs would particularly benefit from regular supervision and contact with other CNSs/NPs from their specialties. Through this activity, the CNSs/NPs will learn from each other by sharing their experiences and ways in which they have resolved difficult situations.

Barriers to clinically effective care are related to disorganisation. Disorganisation is associated with role fragmentation and role confusion. It is recommended that NHS and other healthcare facilities undertake a comprehensive review of all job descriptions of the CNSs and NPs. This should be undertaken collaboratively with CNSs and NPs and that consensus regarding main duties and key tasks occurs so that fragmentation of role function is alleviated.

In relation to Advanced Practice, it is apparent more (for example, assumption of physical assessment skills and diagnosis) could be assumed if barriers to enhancing clinically effective care were resolved. This could be achieved if role clarification occurred. There would be time then for the CNS/NP to extend practice. Regular audits and evaluations of practice would enable role clarification by acknowledging the interventions carried out by the CNS/NP. Regular audits and evaluations of practice would identify areas of practice that need to be improved as well as provide an avenue for recognizing clinically effective care – a view supported in Wilson and Tingle's (1999) paper. The involvement of all CNSs/NPs in audit should be initiated through a clinical governance/shared governance model of nursing (Cox 2000b).

Appendix

Table A3.1 Questionnaire One (Panel of Experts)

'Making a Difference' developing Clinical Effectiveness among Clinical Nurse Specialists (CNS) and Nurse Practitioners (NP)

Overarching Theme = Smoothing the Way Forward

Thematic analysis

- Role confusion
- Negotiation
- Role fragmentation
- Educator
- Professional recognition
- CNS/NP as a Counsellor
- Role development

Please place a tick corresponding to your agreement or disagreement with the following statements:

Role confusion

Role confusion is particularly noticeable in specialties where the CNS/NP has been recently introduced.

We need to educate doctors and other members of the Multi-Disciplinary Team about the role of the CNS and NP.

New nurse specialist roles create role confusion.

Members of the Multi-Disciplinary Team misunderstand the role of the specialist nurse.

The CNS and NP have easily identifiable role boundaries.

Ward staff are deskilled by the CNS and NP.

The ward sisters are the real nurse specialists.

Clear-cut boundaries of care are required to ensure clinically effective care is implemented by CNSs and NPs.

The ward staff perceive CNSs and NPs as an 'extra pair of hands'.

New specialists roles are often a case of trial and error.

The CNS and NP need to demonstrate their clinical credibility before they are recognized as competent CNSs/NPs.

CNSs and NPs only focus on their area of expertise.

The CNSs/NPs can set their own boundaries for practice.

Negotiation

The CNS and NP essentially smooth the way forward in client care because their expertise and knowledge place them in an ideal position to identify potential problems relating to patient care.

The CNS and NP are excellent troubleshooters because their knowledge and expertise enables them to rationalise and recognize patient problems.

CNSs and NPs modify their roles to fit in with the resources available in their Trust.

CNSs and NPs are more autonomous in their clinical decision-making than other nurses/midwives.

Negotiating clinical problems relating to nursing care, is most effectively carried out by the CNSs and NPs, since their expertise and knowledge place them in an ideal position to rationalise the need for a particular intervention.

The role of the CNS and NP is modified and negotiated on a daily basis.

The knowledge and expertise associated with CNSs and NPs places them in an ideal position to negotiate clinical decisions/problems with senior members of the MDT.

Specialist roles involve negotiation of role boundaries on a daily basis.

The CNSs/NPs have more power to influencing decision making than other nurses/midwives.

The CNSs and NPs essentially cause friction in relation to client care because their expertise and knowledge place them in the position to rationalise potential problems relating to patient care.

Role fragmentation

The CNSs and NPs only focus on their area of expertise and do not provide holistic patient care.

CNSs and NPs treat the client holistically.

Fragmentation of the CNSs and NPs is caused by drawing them into issues that are not related to their specialist role.

The ward sisters are the real nurse specialists.

The role of the CNSs and NPs is fragmented because they get involved in non-CNS/NP functions which are not related to their specialist role.

The role of the CNSs and NPs is very isolated.

A lack of resources creates role fragmentation among the CNSs and NPs.

Educator

CNSs and NPs play a key role in supporting junior doctors and nurses in their clinical practice.

CNSs and NPs do not have the time to actively engage in research relating to their field of expertise.

CNSs and NPs play an integral role in educating nurses.

CNSs and NPs play an integral role in educating doctors.

CNSs and NPs are actively engaged in research relating to their field of expertise.

Professional Recognition

Peer support and guidance is necessary for staff development.

The MDT fail to perceive the CNSs/NPs as specialists in their own rights.

The CNSs and NPs are often the first port of call when there are problems relating to the care of a client in their specialist area.

Doctors value the opinion of CNSs and NPs.

Nurses value the opinion of CNSs and NPs.

Doctors often fail to recognize the value and importance of the CNS and NP.

Members of the MDT fail to recognize the value and importance of the CNS and NP.

CNSs/NPs are often approached for advice relating to the care of a patient in their field of expertise.

Clients open up and discuss issues more readily with the CNS/NP than with ward staff.

The CNSs/NPs as a Counsellor

The CNSs/NPs support and guide junior colleagues on a daily basis.

The CNSs/NPs are approached by junior colleagues to 'unload' their daily problems.

The CNSs/NPs maintain a high level of rapport between their colleagues; consequently colleagues confide in them.

Role Development

Clinical supervision is an integral aspect of the development of the CNSs and NPs' roles.

Evaluating patient outcomes through research and clinical audit is a continuous process that all CNSs and NPs are involved in.

The CNSs/NPs do not engage in conducting regular clinical audits, therefore, areas that require improvement in practice suffer neglect.

CNSs and NPs should periodically collaborate with other nurse specialists in their field in order to exchange ideas and improve client care.

Table A3.2 Biographical Questionnaire

Section 1: Information about Yourself

Name:

....

Please give your job title:

....

Please specify which speciality you practice in:

....

Please circle your current grade: F G H I

How long have you been practising as a CNS/NP?

<1 year 1–3 years 3–5 years
5–7 years 7–9 years >10 years

Section 2: Qualifications and Further Study

Please tick the qualifications you have been awarded

Diploma Dip.Ed. BSc. BA
MSc. MA

Please list any other qualifications you have been awarded

....

Are you currently engaged in a course of study? YES NO

If yes, please state the type of course ....

Are you currently engaged in clinical supervision? If yes, please state type of supervision (e.g., group or individual)

....

Table A3.3 Pilot Questionnaire

'Making a Difference' Developing Clinical Effectiveness among Clinical Nurse Specialists (CNS) and Nurse Practitioner's (NP)

Clinical Nurse Specialists and Nurse Practitioners have indicated the following statements either foster or hinder the ability of the specialist nurse to engage in or provide clinically effective care. Please circle the numbers below indicating your agreement or disagreement with the following statements

	Strongly Disagree	*Disagree*	*Agree*	*Strongly Agree*
Role confusion is particularly noticeable in specialties where the CNS/NP has been recently introduced.	1	2	3	4
We need to educate doctors and other members of the multi and disciplinary team about the role of the CNS and NP.	1	2	3	4
The CNS and NP have easily identifiable role boundaries.	1	2	3	4
Ward staff are sometimes deskilled by the CNS and NP.	1	2	3	4
The ward staff sometimes perceive CNSs and NPs as an 'extra pair of hands'.	1	2	3	4
New specialists roles are often a case of trial and error.	1	2	3	4
The CNS and NP need to demonstrate their clinical credibility before they are recognized as competent CNSs/NPs.	1	2	3	4
CNSs and NPs only focus on their area of expertise.	1	2	3	4
The CNSs/NPs can set their own boundaries for practice.	1	2	3	4
The CNS and NP essentially smooth the way forward in client care because their expertise and knowledge place them in an ideal position to identify potential problems relating to patient care.	1	2	3	4
The CNS and NP are excellent troubleshooters because their knowledge and expertise enables them to rationalise and recognize patient problems.	1	2	3	4

Table A3. 3 *contd.*

	Strongly Disagree	*Disagree*	*Agree*	*Strongly Agree*
CNSs and NPs are more autonomous in their clinical decision-making than other nurses/ midwives.	1	2	3	4
Specialist roles involve negotiation of role boundaries on a daily basis.	1	2	3	4
The CNSs/NPs have more power in influencing decision making than other nurses/midwives.	1	2	3	4
The CNS and NP only focus on their area of expertise and do not provide holistic patient care.	1	2	3	4
The role of the CNS and NP is fragmented because they get involved in non CNS/NP functions which are not related to their specialist role.	1	2	3	4
The role of the CNS and NP is very isolated.	1	2	3	4
A lack of resources creates role fragmentation among the CNS and NP.	1	2	3	4
CNSs and NPs play a key role in supporting junior doctors and nurses/midwives in their clinical practice.	1	2	3	4
CNSs and NPs do not have the time to actively engage in research relating to their field of expertise.	1	2	3	4
CNSs and NPs play an integral role in educating nurses/midwives.	1	2	3	4
CNSs and NPs play an integral role in educating doctors.	1	2	3	4
CNSs and NPs are actively engaged in research relating to their field of expertise.	1	2	3	4
Peer support and guidance is necessary for staff development.	1	2	3	4
The CNSs and NPs are often the first port of call when there are problems relating to the care of a client in their specialist area.	1	2	3	4
Doctors value the opinion of CNSs and NPs.	1	2	3	4
Nurses value the opinion of CNSs and NPs.	1	2	3	4
CNS/NPs are often approached for advice relating to the care of a patient in their field of expertise.	1	2	3	4

Clients open up and discuss issues more readily with the CNS/NP than with ward staff.	1	2	3	4
The CNS/NP support and guide junior colleagues on a daily basis.	1	2	3	4
The CNSs/NPs maintain a high level of rapport between their colleagues; consequently colleagues confide in them.	1	2	3	4
Clinical supervision is an integral aspect of the development of the CNSs and NPs roles.	1	2	3	4
Evaluating patient outcomes through research and clinical audit is a continuous process that CNSs and NPs are involved in.	1	2	3	4
The CNSs/NPs do not engage in conducting regular clinical audits; therefore areas that require improvement in practice do not occur.	1	2	3	4
CNSs and NPs should periodically collaborate with other nurse specialists in their field in order to exchange ideas and improve client care.	1	2	3	4

Thank you for completing this questionnaire.

Table A3.4 National Organisation of Nurse Practitioners Framework (NONPF 1995)

The six domains of Advanced Nursing Practice

1. Management of Client Health/Illness Status

- Health promotion/disease prevention: provides anticipatory guidance and counselling regarding wellness, lifestyle, disease risks, and potential changes in health status.
- Develops and analyses appropriate differential diagnoses for presenting client symptoms.

2. The Nurse–Client Relationship

- Creates a relationship, which acknowledges the client's strengths and assists the client in addressing his/her needs.
- Provides emotional and informational support to clients and their families.

3. The Teaching–Coaching Function

- Timing: creates an environment in which effective learning can take place, specifically altering the environment if necessary so that the client can attend to the learning process.
- Monitors the client's behaviour and specific outcomes as a useful guide to evaluating the effectiveness and need to change or maintain teaching strategies.

4. Professional Role

- Functions in a variety of role dimensions: healthcare provider, consultant, educator, administrator and researcher.
- Evaluates implications of contemporary health policy on healthcare providers and consumers.

5. Managing and Negotiating Health Care Delivery Systems

- Provides care for individuals, families, and communities within integrated health care services using nationally accepted guidelines and standards.
- Negotiation: assesses, plans, implements and evaluates health care collaboratively with other healthcare professionals using approaches that recognize each one's expertise and interest to meet the comprehensive needs of clients.

6. Monitoring and Ensuring the Quality of Health Care Practices

- Critically evaluates and applies research studies pertinent to client care management and outcomes.
- Monitors peers, self and delivery system through Quality Assurance, total quality management, as part of continuous quality improvement.

References

Brink, P. and M. Wood (1998) *Advanced Design in Nursing Research*, 2nd edn, London, Sage

Burgess, R. (1982) *Field Research: a sourcebook and field manual*, London, George Allen and Unwin

Castledine, G. (2000a) 'Clinical governance: opportunity for nurses?' *British Journal of Nursing*, 9(10) p. 670

Castledine, G. (2000b) 'Are specialist nurses deskilling general nurses?' *British Journal of Nursing*, 9(11) p. 738

Cox, C. (2000a) 'The Nurse Consultant: An Advanced Nurse Practitioner?' *Nursing Times*, 96(13) p. 48

Cox, Carol L. (2000b) 'Clinical Governance and Shared Governance', *Practice Nursing*, 11(16) pp. 17–20

Cox, C. and Ahluwalia, S. (2000) 'Enhancing Clinical Effectiveness Among Clinical Nurse Specialists', *British Journal of Nursing*, 9(16) pp. 1064–73

Department of Health (1997) *The New NHS Modern and Dependable*, London, HMSO

Department of Health (1998a) *Saving Lives: Our Healthier Nation*, London, HMSO

Department of Health (1998b) *A First Class Service: Quality in the New NHS*, London, HMSO

Department of Health (1999a) *Clinical Governance: Quality in the New NHS*, Leeds, NHSE

Department of Health (1999b) *National Institute for Clinical Excellence*, London, HMSO

Dopson, S., J. Gabbay, J. Locock and D. Chambers (1999) *Evaluation of the PACE Programme: final report*, Oxford Health Care Management Institute, Tempelton College, University of Oxford, Wessex Institute for Health Research and Development, University of Southampton

Hammersley, M. and P. Atkinson (1983) *Ethnography: Principals in Practice*, London, Tavistock

Hammersley, M. and P. Atkinson (1990) *Reading Ethnographic Research: A Critical Guide*, London, Longman

Hicks, C. (1997) 'Research: the dilemma of incorporating research into clinical Practice', *British Journal of Nursing*, 6(9) pp. 511–15

Hinds, P., S. Scandrett-Hibden and L. McCauley (1989) 'Further Assessment of a Method to Estimate Reliability and Validity of Qualitative Research Findings', *Journal of Advanced Nursing*, 15(4) pp. 235–41

Lincoln, Y. and E. Guba (1985) *Naturalistic Enquiry*, California, Sage

Mackenzie, A. (1994) 'Evaluating Ethnography: Considerations for Analysis', *Journal of Advanced Nursing*, 19(4) pp. 774–81

McLaughlin, F. and L. Marasculio (1990) *Advanced Nursing and Health Care Research*, London, W.B. Saunders

Miles, M. and A. Huberman (1994) *An Expanded Source Book: Qualitative Data Analysis*, London, Sage

Morse, J. (1991) *Qualitative Nursing Research: A Contemporary Dialogue*, London, Sage

National Health Service Executive (1996) *Achieving Effective Practice: A clinical effectiveness and research information pack for nurses, midwives and health visitors*, Leeds, NHSE

NONPF (National Organisation of Nurse Practitioners Faculties Curriculum Guidelines Task Force) (1995) *Advanced Nursing Practice, Curriculum Guidelines and Programme Standards for Nurse Practitioner Education*, Washington DC

Polit, D. and B. Hungler (1991) *Nursing Research, Principles and Methods*, 4th edn, London, J.B. Lippincott

Silverman, D. (1993) *Interpreting Qualitative Data*, Gower, Hants, Aldershot

Watson, J. (1999) *Postmodern Nursing and Beyond*, Edinburgh, Churchill Livingstone

Wilson, J. and J. Tingle, (1999) 'Clinical audit systems', *British Journal of Nursing*, 8(12) pp. 821–2

CHAPTER 4

Alteration in Cardiovascular Function: Caring for the Patient with Septic Shock

ANN M. PRICE AND DAWN KAVANAGH

Patient Profile

Mr D. is a 49-year-old Caucasian male who divorced his wife sometime ago. He has two sons with whom he has little contact due to a family dispute. Mr D. stated that he only wished his family to be contacted if his condition was life threatening. He has been unemployed for sometime but leads an independent life. He shares a house with a close friend.

Risk Factors

Mr D. started to drink alcohol excessively after his divorce and now admits to drinking 4 to 6 cans of bitter a day. He has had a peptic ulcer since 1974, which has been managed on oral medication. He also smokes 20 gms of tobacco per day. Despite being advised to reduce or stop his alcohol consumption and smoking he has been unable to achieve this.

Chief Complaint

Mr D. attended the accident and emergency department with a one-day history of severe, constant upper abdominal pain that radiated to his back. He had felt constantly nauseous and vomited blood stained fluid once. He was admitted to hospital and had oversewing of a perforated duodenal ulcer that evening. Following the operation he complained of feeling warm and sweaty and was very thirsty. Nursing diagnosis indicated that he was dehydrated with a chest infection. He experienced an episode of fast atrial fibrillation that was controlled using digoxin. One week after his initial operation his wound started to ooze black fluid and naso-gastric aspiration increased. He was taken to the operating theatre and had drainage of multiple abdominal abscesses and repair of a large duodenal ulcer. Mr D. was admitted to the intensive care unit post-operatively for management of his septicaemia, pneumonia and a large open wound. He was sedated and ventilated and quickly deteriorated into septic shock.

Other Complaints

Pain control was difficult for Mr D.. His large abdominal wound affected his ventilation because he was splinting his respirations. Although he was sedated, his facial expression showed grimacing when the wound site was touched. His analgesia was reviewed and increased and he was paralysed to facilitate ventilation because his hypoxia was increasing. His chest X-ray showed evidence of impending adult respiratory distress syndrome (ARDS).

Definition of the Problem – Pathophysiology

Septic shock 'is a clinically defined entity of altered organ perfusion resulting from systemic response to infection' (Shoenberg *et al.* 1998).

Transmission and Disease Process

Approximately 19 per cent of patients admitted to an intensive care unit suffer from a form of sepsis, systemic inflammatory response syndrome (SIRS) or septic shock. (Shoenberg *et al.* 1998) Mortality rates vary with SIRS being 6–7 per cent and septic shock over 50 per cent (Shoenberg *et al.* 1998). Abdominal sepsis has the highest mortality rate at over 40 per cent according to Wakefield *et al.* (1998) and over 70 per cent according to Shoenberg *et al.* (1998). The long-term prognosis is also poor, with a third of patients not surviving a year after the insult (Shoenberg *et al.* 1998).

Septic shock can be precipitated by a number of mechanisms such as trauma, surgery and pneumonia (Crowley 1996). The infecting organisms may be bacterial, viral, fungal or parasitic. All can lead to the same systemic inflammatory response, which is characteristic of severe sepsis. Gram-negative and gram-positive bacilli are particularly associated with septic shock because of the respective endotoxin and exotoxin release; these activate cellular, hormonal and immunological defences such as cytokines and interlukin 6 (Hudak *et al.* 1998) which results in a self destructive response to the critical insult (Gloris 1999). These processes lead to a distributive form of shock where there is a maldistribution of blood volume (Crowley 1996).

Two main processes involved are in the systemic inflammatory response syndrome:

- Massive vasodilatation results from the loss of vascular responsiveness due to reduced sympathetic stimulation and enhanced production of endothelial derived products (Crowley 1996).
- Intravascular volume is lost due to the leaking capillaries, which results in the development of oedema in vascular beds; this leads to the destruction of vascular endothelium, which contributes to multiple organ dysfunction syndrome (Crowley 1996).

Many of the signs, symptoms and complications of septic shock are a result of these two processes.

Signs and Symptoms

Signs and symptoms of septic shock will vary depending on the severity of the insult, the adequacy of fluid resuscitation, the presence of existing myocardial dysfunction and drugs/treatments used that may affect cardiovascular status (Crowley 1996).

Hudak *et al.* (1998) describes septic shock as a continuum from Hyperdynamic State with high cardiac output, low SVR, hyperpyrexia, polyuria, warm skin and low intravascular volume progressing to a Hypodynamic State as the patient deteriorates. The Hypodynamic State is characterised by low cardiac output, cool skin and oliguria and is opposite to the Hyperdynamic State. Hudak *et al.* (1998) regard the Hypodynamic State as a signal that death is approaching.

Table 4.1 Manifestations of Septic Shock

Clinical Signs	*Invasive Signs (e.g. PAFC, ABGs)*
Hypotension	Low systemic vascular resistance (SVR)
	High pulmonary vascular resistance (PVR)
Tachycardia/ bounding pulse	High or low cardiac output
Tachypnea/ respiratory distress/ hypoxia	Respiratory alkalosis
Temperature (hyper/hypo)	Metabolic acidosis
Warm, flushed or cool, pale skin	Hyper/hypoglycaemia
Altered mental status	Increased or decreased white blood cells
Oliguria/polyuria	*Low PAWP and CVP*

Source: (based on Hudak *et al.* 1998 and American College of Chest Physicians 1997)
Notes: PAFC – pulmonary artery floatation catheter
ABGs – arterial blood gas analysis
PAWP – pulmonary artery wedge pressure
CVP – central venous pressure

Definitions

All of the definitions described in this chapter have been derived from the *American College of Chest Physicians/Society of Critical Care Medicine in Critical Care Medicine* 1997, Vol. 25 No. 11 pp. 790, unless otherwise stated in the text.

- Systemic inflammatory response syndrome – the systemic inflammatory response to a variety of severe clinical insults. The response, is manifested by two or more of the following conditions:
  Temperature >38.0 C or <36.0 C
  Heart rate >90 beats per minute
  Respiratory rate >20 breaths/minute or PaCo2 <32 torr (<4.3 Kpa)
  WBC >12 000 cells/mm3, <4000 ce;s/mm3 or >10 per cent immature (band) forms
- Sepsis – the systemic response to infection. The systemic response is manifested by the same criteria for SIRS.
- Severe sepsis – sepsis associated with organ dysfunction, hypoperfusion, or hypotension. Hypoperfusion and perfusion abnormalities may include, but are not limited to, lactic acidosis, oliguria, or acute alteration in mental status.
- Septic shock – sepsis associated with hypotension despite adequate fluid resuscitation, along with the presence of perfusion abnormalities as listed for severe sepsis. Patients who are on inotropic or vasopressor agents may not be hypotensive at the time that perfusion abnormalities are measured.
- Hypotension – a systolic blood pressure of <90 mmHg or a reduction of >40 mmHg from baseline in the absence of other causes for hypotension.
- Multiple organ dysfunction syndrome – asystolic blood pressure <90 mmHg or a reduction of 40 mmHg from baseline in the absence of other causes of hypotension. Abraham *et al.* (2000) indicated that the definitions described symptoms and did not link to the underlying pathophysiology. This makes it difficult to distinguish the process behind various causes of sepsis.

Treatment

Early recognition of the signs and symptoms of septic shock and appropriate treatment is paramount to survival (Balk 1998). Prompt and aggressive treatment is vital to stabilise the patient when first presenting with septic shock in the intensive care unit.

Table 4.2 Treatment of Septic Shock

Immediate treatment *<6 hours*	*Longer term treatment* *>6 hours*
Broad spectrum antibiotics	Specific antibiotics for the identified infection
Aggressive fluid replacement	Monitor haemodilution, give blood products for Hb and clotting, give fluids according to CVP and PAWP
Vasopressor or inotropic agents to support blood pressure	Titrate inotropes considering CO, SVR, mean arterial BP, SvO2 and urine output
Adequate oxygenation and respiratory support	Risk of ARDS – monitor arterial blood gases and titrate respiratory support
Monitor metabolic environment and renal function	*Initiate nutritional support, control temperature, consider diuretics/renal replacement therapy*

Source: (based on Hudak *et al.* 1998)
Notes: Hb – haemoglobin
CO – cardiac output
BP – blood pressure
SvO2 – mixed venous saturation
ARDS – acute respiratory distress syndrome

Hudak *et al.* (1998) noted that septic shock is a complex process and indicate that a multi-disciplinary approach is needed to treat all the organ systems involved. Treatment revolves around tackling the cause of the septic shock and supporting the organs through a period of poor perfusion to maintain their function.

There have been many research projects examining different treatment, which particularly focus on preventing the damaging effects of endotoxin and cytokines (Protopapas and Mcluckie 1996). However, no one treatment has been proven to be effective in controlling the systemic inflammatory response. This is thought to be due to the complex and multi-factorial biochemical reactions involved (Nystrom 1998).

Domain I – Management of Client Health/Illness Status

Immediate Management

Mr D., upon return from theatre, showed evidence of hypovoleamia with a low CVP and low mean blood pressure and tachycardia. He was aggressively fluid resuscitated using blood products and colloids to replace his intravascular volume as recommended by Meier-Hellman *et al.* (1999). A pulmonary artery catheter was inserted which demonstrated a high cardiac output, low systemic vascular resistance and pyrexia; these were all signs consistent with septic shock. Mr D. was commenced on inotropic support and broad spectrum antibiotics. The inotropic support consisted of a vasoconstriciting agent of noradrenaline to improve his low system vascular resistance (SVR) and adrenaline to improve muscle contractility of the heart thus improving blood pressure. Oliguria was present with a mild metabolic acidosis, which responded well to fluid resuscitation and inotropic support. Mr D. was mechanically ventilated using a pressure-regulated mode on 60 per cent oxygen to maintain good oxygen delivery to the tissues. His initial arterial blood gases were satisfactory. He required sedation using propofol and alfentanyl to facilitate ventilation and control his pain.

Ongoing Management

While Mr D.'s condition improved, his cardiovascular status required constant reassessment including continuous monitoring of cardiac and haemodyanamic parameters to detect early signs of deterioration. Patients with septic shock are at high risk of a number of complications, which require acute observation to detect and treat before multiple organ dysfunction syndrome ensues (Edwards 1993). Skin colour, pulses and temperature give an indication of the effectiveness of the peripheral circulation. The continued recording of pulmonary artery catheter readings allows for prompt fluid resuscitation, which is frequently required as the circulation becomes *leaky* and body water and albumin move into the extravascular space causing oedema. Inotropic support can be adjusted to the individual patient in order to maintain an adequate blood pressure, cardiac output and urine output by examining the systemic vascular resistance and contractility of the heart. Achieving supra normal values is not considered beneficial (Meier-Hellman *et al.* 1999). Mixed venous saturation (SvO2) is recorded to ensure that oxygen delivery to the tissues is maintained so that tissue repair can occur.

Microbiological screening involving all potential sites of infection, for example, sputum, urine, blood and wound cultures were sent to the laboratory in an attempt to isolate the organism responsible for the septic episode. Strict asepsis in all procedures was required to prevent secondary infection particularly in regards to the open abdominal wound. Arterial blood gases were taken to examine the adequacy of ventilation, detect hypoxia and metabolic response to illness. Acute respiratory distress syndrome (ARDS) is a potential complication of critical illness and can be detected by hypoxia and hypercapnia despite adequate ventilation and infiltrates on chest X-ray (Shoenberg *et al.* 1998). ARDS is precipitated by a number of causes and Mr D. had a high risk of developing this complication. Mr D. was placed on a rotational therapy bed to aid prevention of atelectasis and improve ventilation-perfusion (VQ) mismatching. Hyperglycemia is common in these patients and insulin by infusion may be required.

Septic shock leads to a high metabolic rate and increased energy requirements, which demands early nutrition (Nobuya *et al.* 1998). Mr D. was nourished using total parenteral nutrition because he lacked bowel sounds indicating absence of gut motility, and his open abdominal wound meant that he was unable to be fed enterally. This situation was reassessed daily as enteral feeding is the preferred route of nutrition for gut integrity and reduction in translocation of bacteria (Ball 1994).

Mr D. was at risk of disseminated intravascular coagulopathy (DIC) because of the disease process. Assessment of gums, wound, urine, ecchymosis and sputum for signs of bleeding is essential in addition to monitoring of clotting studies to detect deterioration and treat as necessary. In extreme circumstances DIC can lead to intracerebral and gastrointestinal bleeding which can be fatal (Hudak *et al.* 1998). Therefore, close monitoring using the Glasgow Coma Score for assessment of neurological function, regular nasogastric aspiration for blood and monitoring for sudden drops in haemoglobin to detect early signs of bleeding should be performed by the CNS.

Pressure area care is vital to maintain skin integrity. Regular moving, avoiding shearing forces and maintaining hygiene to keep the skin clean and dry is important in the maintenance of skin integrity.

Domain II – The Nurse–Client Relationship

Immediate Management

Mr D. experienced a high level of pain and discomfort from his large open wound and the many invasive lines attached to him, which he demonstrated through his facial expressions although he was unable to talk because he was intubated endotracheally. He also demonstrated tachycardia, which increased during procedures such as suctioning, mouth, and pressure area care. It was difficult for the CNS to assess whether his reactions were due to pain or anxiety because he was unable to express his feelings and so both aspects were addressed. Analgesia was given and his response assessed and he was verbally reassured, orientated to time and place, and procedures were explained to him prior to commencement. Non-verbal communication was used to display caring, such as holding his hand, alongside gentle verbal encouragement (Leng and Lawson 1998).

Ongoing Management

Mr D. had been estranged from his wife and sons for four years and he had expressed the wish that they were not to be contacted unless his condition was life threatening. As his condition was extremely serious it was deemed appropriate to contact his family. Establishing contact was difficult as the contact number on Mr D.'s records was incorrect. The police were asked to make additional contacts to notify the next of kin of Mr D.'s hospitalisation. When the family visited they did not know how to react because they had not had contact with Mr D. for a long time. The sons particularly found it difficult because they were confused about the relationship they had with their father. Counselling was suggested for the sons using the bereavement service available in the hospital. The sons' interaction with their father was allowed to take a natural course so as not to cause undue distress but to support them as necessary.

Mr D. suffered from an altered body image due to his large open abdominal wound and potential role identity crisis regarding his relationship with his sons. The CNS was aware this might lead to feelings of isolation and consequential depression. This cannot be prevented, but may be alleviated by being aware of potential feelings and confusion he may experience. The CNS assured him that his wound would heal and that she would discuss methods of disguising the scar when he felt better. The relationship with his sons was difficult. It was recognized Mr D. may not wish to re-establish a relationship with them. Therefore, he required counselling once he had made a decision, whatever that would be. The CNS offered the support, reassurance and guidance he needed.

Mr D. was at risk of developing intensive care psychosis, which is demonstrated through hallucinations, restlessness and sleep impairment. The environment was adjusted to allow for periods of rest and sleep to promote a normal biorthymn. Sedation was reduced when his condition was stable so that he could be fully orientated to his surroundings, establish a daily routine and allow interaction with the people around him.

Domain III – The Teaching Coaching Function

Immediate Management

Initially post-operatively Mr D. was not alert and could not process any information regarding health promotion at this stage.

The focus for the Clinical Nurse Specialist during this episode is to ensure that staff are aware of the signs and symptoms and treatment regime for septic shock. One nurse said that she was not happy using the cardiac output studies machine. The machine's functions were explained to the nurse and the process of collecting data demonstrated. She was observed collecting the data and the findings were discussed with the CNS. This allowed for a discussion regarding Mr D.'s condition and treatment and changes that might be required depending on the cardiac output results. Examples were given regarding possible readings and preferred treatments were discussed. Mr D.'s readings were examined and the nurse subsequently suggested a treatment regime, which was implemented.

Ongoing Management

When Mr D. was able to discuss his lifestyle, appropriate guidance regarding his alcohol intake and smoking were given. The CNS knew that critically ill patients are often unaware of the seriousness of their illness or the life-threatening condition that they have been in (Wesson 1997). Gentle but honest information regarding his illness can lead to a discussion about how to prevent its reoccurrence.

Staff education and support concerning septic patients is vital to improve knowledge and relate theory to practice. Education can be managed in a number of ways, such as formal and informal teaching sessions, ward rounds, multi-disciplinary case study presentations and supervised clinical experience. Reflection is encouraged, using a clinical supervision framework, so that staff can learn from the experiences of caring for Mr D. and utilise the knowledge for similar patients on future occasions (Price and Chalker 2000).

Domain IV – Professional Role

Immediate Management

Part of the CNS role is to demonstrate proactive leadership both in caring for the patient and his family and acting as an expert adviser for staff. For example, a rotational therapy bed was recommended by the CNS, on the multi-disciplinary ward round, because she was aware of Mr D.'s potential risk of developing ARDS. The consultant anesthetist immediately agreed with this course of action and the treatment bed was ordered.

The availability and approachability of the Clinical Nurse Specialist is important to act as a role model and to actively give advice and support as required to staff. A junior doctor will often seek advice to reassure him/herself that every aspect of care has been covered. The CNS was questioned regarding Mr D.'s temperature regulation, which remained high. The CNS confirmed that the doctor had already taken blood cultures and reviewed the antibiotic regimen. It was suggested that the doctor contact the microbiologist for further advice on the patient's management.

Ongoing Management

The CNS needs to keep abreast of the ongoing developments with Mr D.'s treatment, family and other issues, to ensure that a holistic approach to care is maintained. A team nursing approach can be utilised to ensure continuity of care and good communication between all members of the multi-disciplinary team. The CNS also ensures documentation of the changes in Mr D.'s management is accurately recorded by the multi-disciplinary team.

Domain V – Managing and Negotiating Health Care Delivery Systems

Immediate Management

The CNS is based within the intensive care unit and is, therefore, readily available to offer advice and guidance to staff and students. The nurse specialist cares for patients on the intensive care unit so that his/her skills can be used to full advantage to benefit patient care.

Ongoing Management

The CNS has a duel role within the intensive care unit, that of manager and clinical specialist. The Newham General Hospital ITU, like many other hospital ITUs, has a high demand for its intensive care beds. Sometimes demand outweighs supply. The CNS in this unit has been involved in developing admission and discharge criteria to ensure that patients are not admitted inappropriately. The CNS ensures that the correct procedures and criteria are followed for admitting patients to the unit. In addition, the CNS monitors admission and discharge of patients through audit as recommended in national guidelines (DoH 2000).

Domain VI – Monitoring and Ensuring the Quality of Health Care Practice

Immediate Management

Friedman *et al.* (1998) noted that mortality rates for septic shock have improved slightly and attributed this to an increase in gram-positive as opposed to gram-negative septicemia. Abdominal sepsis continues to have one of the poorest prognoses (Friedman *et al.* 1998) and, thus, Mr D.'s long-term survival is not guaranteed. This can highlight some ethical dilemmas for staff in regard to the futility of treatment in the event of his deterioration. Two main issues were noted, the fact that Mr D. was in a degree of discomfort despite large amounts of analgesia and his poor prognosis considering his multiple problems. The ethical debate focused on inflicting unnecessary suffering on Mr D. However, Mr D. was responding positively to treatment and had not deteriorated into multi-organ failure.

Ongoing Management

Auditing within the intensive care setting is becoming more important with the introduction of clinical governance and clinically effective practice. Intensive care units need to compare outcomes with each other, share findings and knowledge and utilize this information to develop best practice. Maintaining the knowledge of staff within the intensive care unit is needed to promote innovative and proactive care. The CNS ensures that learning needs are facilitated and that best practice is provided at all times. The CNS undertakes regular audits of nursing care and reviews protocols and guidelines to ensure high standards of practice are achieved.

The level of research undertaken within intensive care units is often small and isolated. Intra-unit collaboration can establish good lines of communication. The CNS can facilitate and encourage research activities. A Nursing Critical Care Forum has been developed within the wider London area by CNSs in order to share developments, research findings and innovative practice. Its activities are intended to aid communication and stimulate change within intensive care units throughout the London area.

References

Abraham, E., M. Mathay, C. Dinarello, J. Vincent, J. Cohen, S. Opal, M. Glauser, P. Parsons, C. Fisher and J. Repine (2000) 'Consensus conference definitions for sepsis, septic shock, acute lung injury and acute respiratory distress syndrome: time for reevaluation', *Critical Care Medicine*, 28,(1) pp. 232–5

Balk, R. (1998) 'Outcome of Septic Shock: Location, location, location', *Critical Care Medicine*, 25(6) pp. 983–4

Ball, C. (1994) 'Intestinal barrier failure and the development of the systemic inflammatory response syndrome', *Intensive and Critical Care Nursing*, 10(4) pp. 252–6

Crowley, F. (1996) 'The Pathogenesis of Septic Shock', *Heart and Lung*, 25(2) pp. 124–34

DoH (2000) *Comprehensive Critical Care: A review of adult critical care services*, Department of Health, London, HMSO

Edwards, J. (1993) 'Management of Septic Shock', *British Medical Journal*, 306(6893) pp. 1661–4

Friedman, G., E. Silva and J. Vincent (1998) 'Has the Mortality Rate with Septic Shock Changed with Time?' *Critical Care Medicine*, 26(12) pp. 2078–86

Gloris, R. (1999) 'Local versus systemic inflammatory responses in shock, trauma and sepsis', *International Journal of Intensive Care*, 6(3) pp. 81–4, 88, 92

Hudak, C., B. Gallo and P. Morton (1998) 'Hypoperfusion Studies', in C. Hudak, B. Gallo and P. Morton (eds) *Critical Care Nursing: A holistic approach*, 7th edn, London, J.B. Lippincott Company

Leng, C. and A. Lawson (1998) 'Pain Management in Intensive Care', in A. Adams and J. Cashman (eds) *Anaesthesia and Analgesia*, Edinburgh, Churchill Livingstone

Meier-Hellman, A., S. Sokra and K. Reinhart (1999) 'Use of Catecholamines in Sepsis', *International Journal of Intensive Care*, 6(4) pp. 118, 120, 122, 125–6

Nobuya, I., L. Plank, K. Sando and G. Hill (1998) 'Optimal Protein Requirements During the First Two Weeks After the Onset of Critical Illness', *Critical Care Medicine*, 26(9) pp. 1529–39

Nystrom, P. (1998) 'The systemic inflammatory response syndrome: definitions and aetiology', *The British Society for Antimicrobial Chemotherapy*, Number 41, Supplement A, pp. 1–7

Price, A. and M. Chalker (2000) 'Our Journey With Clinical Supervision in an Intensive Care Unit', *Intensive and Critical Care Nursing*, 16(1) pp. 51–5

Protopapas, M. and A. McLuckie (1996) 'Sepsis in the Intensive Care Unit', *Care of the Critically Ill*, January/February, 12(1) pp. 21–4

Shoenberg, M., M. Weis and P. Radermacher (1998) 'Outcome of Patients with Sepsis and Septic Shock After ITU Treatment', *Langenbecks Arch Surgery*, 383(1) pp. 44–88

Wakefield, C., G. Barclay, K. Fearon, A. Goldie, J. Ross, I. Grant, A. Ramsay and J. Mowie (1998) 'Proinflammatory mediator activity, endogenous antagonists and the systemic inflammatory response in intra-abdominal sepsis', *British Journal of Surgery*, 85(6) pp. 818–25

Wesson, J. (1997) 'Meeting the Informational, Psychosocial and Emotional needs of each ICU Patient and Family', *Intensive and Critical Care Nursing*, 13(2) pp. 111–18

Chapter 5

Alteration in Respiratory Function: Caring for the Patient with Tuberculosis (TB)

Virginia Gleissberg and Rebecca Hall

Patient Profile

Mr E. was born in St Andrew's Hospital in 1931 and has lived in the East End of London all his life. He is a 68 year old Caucasian male and, although no longer practising, describes himself as Christian. A builder by trade, he retired six years ago and lives with his wife, enjoying frequent contact with his two daughters and three grandchildren who live nearby. He sees his son less often since he went to live in Scotland four years ago.

Risk Factors

Despite smoking 30–40 cigarettes per day since his teenage years, Mr E. described himself as feeling fit up until his late fifties when he started to experience heart problems. At the age of 58 he reduced his smoking to 15 per day and at the age of 62 he took early retirement due to angina. Subsequent to early retirement he has been receiving treatment for depression.

Chief Complaint

Mr E. has had an eight-week history of productive cough, which is worse than his usual smoker's cough. He has also lost his appetite, as well as weight (approximately 5kg in the last month), and is lethargic with occasional sweating during the night. He delayed seeing his GP, as he was worried that his symptoms may be indicative of lung cancer. When he did eventually go to see him he was prescribed antibiotics for a presumed chest infection but made no improvement. One evening he became very short of breath and was complaining of chest pain. His wife, fearing that it had something to do with his heart complaint, became very concerned and took him to accident and emergency at Newham General Hospital. A chest x-ray revealed bilateral shadowing indicative of TB. Therefore he was admitted into an isolation room with full respiratory precautions.

Other Complaints

Having been reassured that he did not have lung cancer, Mr E. became concerned about his infectious state, as well as the stigma attached to his disease. He found it difficult to adjust to being isolated and his mental health deteriorated. Referral was made to the mental health team. His angina remained well controlled. He needed a great deal of support in the early stages of his treatment but became more confident as his condition began to improve.

Definition of the Problem – Pathophysiology

Tuberculosis is a disease caused by *mycobacterium* tuberculosis. Although it can occur anywhere in the body it usually affects the lungs.

Transmission and Disease Process

The host is infected by inhaling airborne droplet nuclei containing tubercle bacilli which have been released into the air as a result of the coughing, sneezing, laughing, talking or singing of someone with active infectious TB. Patients who have the disease in their lungs or larynx are the most infectious as the damage TB causes to the body's tissues gives infectious material direct access to the air. Once inhaled, the bacilli usually remain within the lungs but may be transported by the blood or via the lymphatic system to other parts of the body.

A body in reasonably good health can usually cope with this by producing antibodies to fight the infection. The host will have no knowledge that this has occurred unless tuberculin testing (heaf or mantoux) is carried out. Someone who is merely infected with TB cannot transmit the disease but, once infected, the host has a 10 per cent, that is 1 in 10, chance of going on to develop active disease at any time in their lifetime (Crofton 1992). For those also infected with HIV this chance increases to 50 per cent (O'Brien 1998). The risk of developing active disease increases among highly vulnerable hosts and is even more likely the greater the amount of bacilli inhaled (Crofton 1992).

Contact tracing is a vital part of TB control. Studies have shown that that 10 per cent of TB cases are found through the screening of contacts (Kumar *et al.*

1992; Ormerod 1993). This has been demonstrated by an audit of TB cases in the Borough of Newham in the first four months of 1999. The Joint Tuberculosis Committee (JTC) of the British Thoracic Society (BTS) provides guidance with regard to contact tracing (JTC 994) and stresses that the focus of screening should be on those at highest risk, that is, contacts of pulmonary and, in particular, open pulmonary TB (Leitch 1992).

Signs and symptoms

Signs and symptoms vary according to the site and severity of the disease, however, they will generally include a combination of three or more as shown in Table 5.1. An active case of TB is reflected in an individual with symptomatic disease due to infection with tubercle bacilli. TB cases are classified as either pulmonary or extra-pulmonary. Cases of pulmonary TB are further subdivided into sputum smear- positive and smear-negative according to the results of microscopic examination of sputa. The term smear positive, also known as open TB, refers to a patient who has so many TB bacilli in their sputum that they show up under a microscope when a Ziehl Nielsen and/or auramine (fluorescent) stain is performed. This means that they are much more infectious than someone whose sputum has had to be sent for culture in order to find the bacilli. Although there are a number of mycobacterial infections, which can be identified by the presence of acid-fast bacilli (AFB), when found in sputum the diagnosis is most likely to be TB (Ormerod 1998).

Ideally it is necessary to send three specimens of sputum for AFB investigation, collected on three consecutive days. ‘A single specimen of sputum will miss about 25 per cent of microscopically positive and about 50 per cent of culture positive cases (Jenkins 1998: 71)’. Smear positive patients tend to have

Table 5.1 Signs and Symptoms of Tuberculosis

Pulmonary	*General*
Productive cough	Weight loss
Localised chest pain	Night sweats
Breathlessness	Fever
Haemoptysis	Lethargy
	Fatigue
	Pain at affected area
	Loss of appetite

Source: Humphries and Lam 1998; Ormerod 1998.

more advanced disease with more damage to their lungs so they cough up much more infectious material. Without chemotherapy, the outcome of their disease is poorer than that of smear negative patients, as 50 per cent of them die within five years. Although 30 per cent may recover spontaneously, 20 per cent will continue to be smear positive and, by definition, highly infectious to others (Grzybowski 1991). Smear-negative patients and non-pulmonary cases must also be given chemotherapy if the presence of active TB is likely.

Definitions

- Smear-positive – TB in a patient with at least *two* initial sputum smear examinations positive for Acid Fast Bacilli (AFB +) by direct microscopy;
  Or: TB in a patient with one sputum specimen AFB + and radiographic abnormalities consistent with active pulmonary TB;
  Or: TB in a patient with one sputum specimen AFB + and culture positive for tubercle bacilli.
- Smear-negative – TB in a patient with symptoms suggestive of TB (see Table 5.1) and at least three sputum examinations negative for AFB, and with radiographic abnormalities consistent with active pulmonary TB, followed by a decision to treat the patient with a full course of antituberculosis therapy. A smear negative case whose result is later found to be positive remains *classified* as smear negative.

Microbiological investigation is extremely valuable in the management of TB. It can determine whether or not a patient is infectious; confirm the diagnosis by identifying the specific mycobacteria grown on culture; and measure sensitivities to the drugs being used to treat the disease.

Treatment

TB bacteria behave in a number of different ways, which is why a combination of drugs, with a variety of bactericidal and sterilising actions, is needed to treat the disease effectively (Chan and Yew 1998). For example, there may be actively multiplying bacteria in the cavities, which cause the sputum to be positive; slowly multiplying bacteria in the body defence cells (macrophages) close to the open cavity; and bacteria in solid lesions that divide only intermittently. Five drugs are currently being recommended by the JTC in the treatment of TB (JTC 1998): isoniazid (H), rifampicin (R), pyrazinamide (Z) and ethambutol (E) or streptomycin (S).

Treatment is divided into two phases. The initial intensive phase consists of three or four drugs given daily for at least two months. This rapidly improves clinical symptoms and reduces the bacterial population and sputum positivity without allowing the development of drug resistance. A second, continuation phase consisting of a combination of two drugs aims to eliminate remaining bacilli and prevent subsequent relapse. Patients may be discharged following an uninterrupted six-month course of treatment for fully sensitive TB, as relapse is rare (JTC 1998).

Side effects are uncommon but the patient should be advised to report any skin rashes, jaundice, visual disturbances, impaired hearing, gastro-intestinal problems or tingling in the fingers and toes. Chemotherapy should be interrupted only if severe drug intolerance occurs. This usually involves liver problems as all the most commonly used drugs are hepato-toxic (Chan and Yew 1998). Nausea and mild rashes are the most common reactions and although it is not necessary to alter the regimen it is important to offer support to the patient and prescribe anti-histamines or anti-emetics if necessary. Nausea can often be eliminated or minimised if the medication is taken at the end rather than at the beginning of the day.

The process by which Rifampicin is metabolised can in turn effect the metabolism of a number of other drugs leading potentially to toxicity or drug failure (Grange *et al.* 1994). Among others, oral contraceptives will no longer be effective; epilepsy may no longer be controllable with phenytoin; and opioids will have a reduced effect that can lead to mental health problems being exacerbated (Winstanley 1998). It is important to counsel people as to any other medication they are taking or may need to take during the course of their TB treatment.

Drug Resistance and How it Occurs

There will be more than 10 million bacteria in the actively multiplying bacterial population. In such a vast number there will always be a few bacteria that will be resistant to any one of the anti-TB drugs (Winstanley 1998). Thus, if only one drug is used, a population of bacteria resistance to this drug will develop. If more than one drug is used, any bacteria resistant to one drug will be dealt with by the other drugs. If the drugs are taken irregularly or stopped prematurely drug resistance can occur. The greatest cause of drug resistance is partial adherence – particularly where the patient takes only one of the active drugs prescribed (Chan and Yew 1998). This has serious consequences not only for the individual patient but also for TB control in general. There are, however, many reasons why a patient may not receive adequate treatment including prescription error, dispensing error, unclear information, misunderstanding by the patient, lack of trust, or refusal to take medication. Many of these problems can be recognized and overcome through the development of therapeutic nurse–patient relationships.

Drug resistant TB is difficult to manage, expensive and, in some cases, impossible to cure. The patient may, therefore, remain infectious and spread drug resistant TB in the community.

Planned outcome

The planned outcome for Mr E. is to make a full recovery. The TB clinical nurse specialist (CNS) can usually be confident in her optimism that this goal will be reached as the cure rate is normally very high.

Domain I – Management of Client Health/Illness Status

Immediate Management

The fact that the chest x-ray showed extensive shadowing with evidence of cavitation suggested that Mr E. had pulmonary TB. It was necessary to admit him into respiratory isolation and order three sputum specimens to be sent to the laboratory for AFB investigation. This was done to find out first, whether or not Mr E. was infectious, and second to confirm a diagnosis and establish the organism's sensitivity to the prescribed medications.

Mr E. was started on quadruple chemotherapy by the chest consultant, based on his symptoms and the appearance of the x-ray. The CNS was informed. The following day the CNS received a telephone call from the microbiology laboratory informing her that Mr E.'s sputum was smear positive. That afternoon the CNS visited the patient in the isolation room on the ward to discuss his diagnosis and treatment as well as the contact screening that would have to be arranged. The CNS also organised the official notification of the disease, as required, to the local environmental health department by ensuring that the notification form was filled in accurately and signed by the appropriate doctor.

'Successful control depends on accurate knowledge of the local epidemiology of the disease' (DoH 1996), therefore, the notification of *all* cases of TB is a legal requirement. Anyone who is considered to need treatment for TB should be notified. If, with further investigation, TB turns out not to be the diagnosis, that person can be denotified. Notification of infectious diseases is often the doctor's responsibility, however, the fact that the CNS aims to provide care to all TB patients from the time they are diagnosed gives them the ideal opportunity to organise notification of TB. There is evidence to suggest that this system improves the rate of notification (Pym *et al*, 1995).

Ongoing Management

Mr E. responded well to treatment while in hospital, although he felt quite nauseous for a few hours after taking the medication. He was discharged from hospital two weeks later feeling physically stronger and his nausea had subsided. The CNS visited him at home a week after he had been discharged. During this visit, Mr E. said that he felt a bit flat at not being able to get about very much but that he was feeling reasonably well. He did report a loss of appetite, which he felt was due to the tablets. The CNS advised him that this was not unusual and that he should try to eat a little bit of food often. He should contact her if this continued to be a problem.

The chest consultant was satisfied with Mr E.'s condition when he saw him in the chest clinic two weeks after his discharge from hospital. The CNS made a number of home visits (as described in more detail below) at the request of Mr E. and his family. Although Mr E. had a few problems to start with, by the time he attended for his next review at the chest clinic, two months following the beginning of his treatment, he had gained 2 kgs in weight and was feeling much better.

The microbiology laboratory staff had identified the mycobacteria found in the original sputum sample as tuberculosis and had found the organism to be fully sensitive to all the drugs that had been prescribed. This information, together with the fact that Mr E.'s chest x-ray was showing improvement and that he was gaining weight and generally feeling better, led to his medication being changed from quadruple therapy to dual therapy. He was treated dually with rifampicin and isoniazid.

Mr E. was seen the following month at home by the CNS. He required more than the routine monthly visits to support him through the last few months of treatment. At the final review by the chest consultant, the chest x-ray showed great improvement but residual scarring left him with a slight chest tightness and occasional cough. He was discharged from clinic with open an invitation to self-refer via the TB nurse specialist if he was concerned about his health.

Domain II – The Nurse–Client Relationship

Immediate Management

The CNS visited Mr E. when he was an inpatient two days following his admission. She offered advice and support with regard to his diagnosis and potentially infectious state. As well as discussing various aspects of the disease and its treatment, the CNS offered written materials to reinforce the information given. She gave Mr E. the opportunity to discuss his condition with his family. The local TB nursing service was described and contact telephone numbers were left with an open invitation for either him or family members to use them. Mr E. was at the same time reassured that his condition could only be discussed with his permission.

At this stage it was important to assess Mr E.'s response to the diagnosis with regard to any implications this may have on his treatment. He was pessimistic about his chances of recovery, angry about the fact that he had TB and blamed his Asian neighbours. He was worried about his contact with other family members, especially his granddaughter, as he did not want to *spread* his infection to others.

The CNS acknowledged the difficulties associated with a diagnosis such as TB but reassured Mr E. that the medication available is very effective. The CNS also stressed the fact that he would no longer be infectious after two weeks of treatment (JTC 1998) at which time he would be able to go home. Apart from taking time to recover Mr E. could go about his business as usual. The important thing was to complete his treatment. This could best be achieved by fitting it into his daily routine (Hunt *et al.* 1989).

Initial discussions regarding contact tracing, particularly with regard to social contacts, concerned Mr E., as he did not want people to know that he had TB. He was reassured that his confidentiality would be maintained. Contact tracing was then arranged and close family were seen in the clinic within three weeks of Mr E.'s diagnosis. His granddaughter and one of his daughters were found to be infected with TB and given three months preventive therapy consisting of rifampicin and isoniazid (O'Brien 1998). His social contacts were invited by letter to attend for screening with no mention as to whom they had been in contact with. Screening was arranged for his son at a local Scottish chest clinic. Records were kept as to who was invited for screening, who attended and what the outcomes were. While number of his social contacts were curious as to whom they had had contact with, it was possible to maintain Mr E.'s confidentiality. Appropriate verbal and written information was offered to family members and other contacts about various aspects of the disease.

One week following Mr E.'s admission, the CNS was called to the ward as a result of a confrontation between Mr E. and one of the nurses. The conversation between Mr E. and the CNS revealed that he had previously been receiving treatment for depression and was currently feeling very low due to his condition and the need for him to be isolated. This situation is discussed at greater length in ongoing management of care.

Ongoing Management

The relationship between Mr E. and his wife appeared strained during their interaction. Mrs E. confided that she was angry that he had not sought help earlier; he had been finding his depression difficult to cope with. Mrs E. was particularly annoyed that their daughter and granddaughter had been infected and felt that this could have been avoided. Beneath her anger was extreme concern and a feeling of helplessness in the face of her husband's illness.

A week later Mr E.'s daughter telephoned the CNS, as she was worried about how depressed her father seemed and how little he was eating. The CNS was also concerned about her mother who was having difficulty coping with Mr E.'s illness and more importantly his attitude towards it. A telephone call to Mr E. revealed that he was feeling quite low and that he could not bear his wife nagging him to eat all the time. The CNS arranged another home visit and, with Mr E.'s consent, arranged for both his wife and his daughter to be present. At this visit all were encouraged to talk about their concerns and frustrations.

This was a useful opportunity to discern that, although Mrs E.'s intentions were good, it was unrealistic to expect Mr E. to eat three cooked meals a day. It was decided that it would be better to provide the sort of food that Mr E. might like which could be prepared easily for the time being. It was also decided that Mr E. would set realistic targets for himself in terms of going out. Part of his frustration had arisen because he was unable to go out as he used to do, and the fact that he became very tired when he did so. He therefore decided to limit himself to short walks to a nearby park or café and to gradually do more as he became stronger. The CNS saw Mr and Mrs E. the following week at the chest clinic when Mr E. attended his outpatient appointment with the chest consultant. They both said that things had improved a little and appeared more relaxed. However Mr E. continued to exhibit frustration with his slow progress.

Domain III – The Teaching Coaching Function

Patient

Immediate Management

Mr E. was quite vocal regarding his theory of how he contracted TB. He blamed 'the immigrants' as there are many Asian families living in his area. This required careful discussion including the history of TB in Britain and how common it used to be as recently as the 1950s (Davies 1998). Information about the transmission of TB and how it can lie dormant in the body for many years finally convinced him that he may indeed have been infected during the war and that he was suffering a re-activation.

It is important to find a balance between reassuring the patient that his disease is treatable while maintaining a sufficient level of concern to motivate him to take the treatment for the necessary six-month period. The CNS gave Mr E. a description of potential side effects associated with the drugs used to treat TB, reassured him that severe side effects are rare and stressed the need for problems to be reported in good time.

Ongoing Management

The CNS offered support to Mr E. and his family (particularly his wife) during home visits as well as through telephone contact. It was important to speak to Mr and Mrs E. separately, as well as together, in order that fears and anxieties could be expressed.

Four months after his treatment had begun, Mr E. informed the CNS, during a routine home visit, that he planned to stop taking the tablets. He said that he felt 'back to normal apart from having a bit of a cough' and that the tablets 'interfered' with his life. The CNS reiterated the importance of completing the six-month course to minimise the possibility of relapse and avoid developing drug resistance. After some time Mr E. agreed to continue and the CNS arranged to visit again the following week. The number of tablets that Mr E. still had was recorded which was routine on a home visit and the importance of completing the course was also discussed with Mrs E. After the next visit the CNS visited fortnightly up until the end of Mr E.'s treatment. By this time she was confident, through tablet monitoring and discussions with Mr and Mrs E. that he had adhered to the regimen prescribed.

At the end of treatment it was important for the CNS to ensure that Mr E. understood that, although unlikely to experience problems with TB in the future, it was necessary for him to report any suspicious symptoms early and that he could do that simply by contacting the CNS directly.

Nursing staff and other agencies

Immediate management

When visiting Mr E. on the ward, the CNS ensured that appropriate isolation procedures had been implemented. Mr E. commented that hardly any of the staff spent any time at all with him and he felt like a 'leper'. The CNS contacted the staff nurse who was allocated to care for Mr E. and discussed this issue with her. The CNS asked the nurse to reassure her colleagues that the dust mist respirator masks provided effective protection against infection (Nicas 1995; Willeke and Qian 1998). It was acknowledged that staff on the ward were extremely busy, however respiratory isolation could be socially isolating for a patient. Part of caring for someone in respiratory isolation involves discussing how they are coping and assessing their needs in relation to their enforced environment as much as to their particular health problem (Mayho 1988).

Ongoing management

The CNS gives teaching sessions to a number of different staff groups, both within the hospital and in the local community, with the aim of raising general awareness to encourage appropriate management as well as to reduce the stigma and misunderstanding often associated with TB. Improving relations with local housing, welfare and education staff as well as with healthcare providers can improve the services offered to people suffering with TB who are often the most vulnerable (Moore-Gillon 1998)

Domain IV – Professional Role

Immediate Management

The incident for which the CNS had been called to the ward involved an argument between Mr E., who wanted to go for a smoke, and a nurse who would not allow him out of his isolation room. Mr E. had been quite abusive toward the nurse and she in turn was extremely upset. The CNS discussed the incident at length with Mr E., offering him plenty of time to talk about how he was feeling as well as explaining the need for his isolation and the reason behind the nurse's behaviour. He was angry initially, but calmed down, finally admitting that he did not really want a cigarette. However, he was finding his isolation extremely difficult to cope with.

Mr E. explained that he was feeling very depressed and was worried about this as he had been treated for depression previously. The CNS asked for the details of the mental health physician he used to see as an outpatient. It was agreed that the TB nurse specialist would refer Mr E. to the appropriate team in order that they could review him while he was in hospital. Mr E. was reassured that the review would simply involve an assessment of his current mental state. The chest consultant was informed of the situation by the CNS, who also spoke with, and wrote a referral letter to, the mental health team.

Before leaving the ward the CNS also spoke to the nurse involved in the incident, reassured her that she had indeed been correct in preventing Mr E. from leaving his room. However the situation was more complex and that Mr E. was particularly vulnerable and upset at this time. This must be considered in relation to his past history of depression.

Ongoing Management

The referral to the mental health team led to Mr E. being kept under review as an outpatient. Although he appeared quite low in mood, on occasion, during home visits he had been reassured that his mental state was within normal limits for someone in his situation. He informed the CNS that, if necessary he would visit his GP and obtain anti-depressants, as the psychiatrist had already written to him and recommended this course of action if necessary. He was reluctant, however, to start taking anti-depressants again because of how they made him feel; he had been very glad to come off them two years ago.

Domain V – Managing and Negotiating Health Care Delivery Systems

Immediate Management

The flexibility afforded to the CNS working with patients in the hospital as well as at home provides the patient continuity of care and helps to ensure that the care offered by others is appropriate. This has been described in the examples of the patients experience on the hospital ward.

Ongoing Management

Resource management is an issue in relation to the TB service which must be addressed if TB is to be managed as is recommended by the JTC (1994) and the Department of Health (1996). A major problem is that levels of TB in Newham have risen by 20 per cent in the last five years. This problem is not peculiar to Newham alone. The TB service is intended to be managed according to the to JTC (1994) guidelines which recommend that there be one CNS for every 50 annual notifications. Newham has provision for two and 185 cases of TB were notified in 1998. The growing concern that contact tracing may be inadequate highlighted the need to prioritise restricted resources.

An audit was carried out by the TB nurses to investigate the outcomes of new entrant and contact screening undertaken at Newham Chest Clinic between 1 January 1999 and 30 April 1999. While the results indicated the value of screening new entrants, the fact that insufficient contacts were being traced due to the unmanageable workload of the two TB CNSs, made it a lower priority.

The CNS presented the results of the audit to both the chest physicians and the Consultant of Communicable Disease Control (CCDC) from the local Public Health Department and priorities for the TB service were negotiated. The audit identified resources had to be prioritised to improve contact tracing at the expense of new entrant screening, as the risk of both TB infection and active disease was demonstrably higher in contacts of known TB cases. As well as this making the workload of the TB nurses more manageable, it was an effective way of highlighting the need for increased resources for the service in general.

Domain VI – Monitoring and Ensuring the Quality of Health Care Practice

Immediate Management

Each patient, including Mr E., has an individual record kept by the CNS. As well as standard patient details, a contemporaneous account is made in the records to promote continuity of care. Although patients are allocated to one of two TB nurse specialists according to where they live, there are often occasions when one will have to cover the other's caseload. Alongside the notification system is an enhanced surveillance programme which aims to keep a large amount of epidemiological information on a national database in order to assess local and national trends in tuberculosis. This information is collected by the CNS early on in a patient's course of treatment. A purely local database keeps a record of the outcomes of all those started on treatment. The TB service itself is based on BTS (1994) and DOH (1996) guidelines.

Ongoing Management

Audit is a useful tool to assess activities and identify priorities to make best use of restricted resources. Standards have also been set in view of the current problems facing the service in terms of providing the safest service with the highest possible quality. For instance, prior to the audit described, it was acknowledged that neither new entrant screening nor contact tracing were being satisfactorily implemented. The audit demonstrated that while improvements could be made in both areas, contacts had to take priority as the group at greatest risk from TB. Contact screening will be re-audited during the same period in the years that follow to establish if any changes have occurred.

As well as discussing these issues within the local health institutions, the TB CNSs have been participating in a number of media activities including interviews for local and national newspapers, television and radio. The CNSs always seeks permission from the Healthcare Trust beforehand and are very careful to simply highlight the issue without apportioning blame.

References

Chan, B. and W. Yew (1998) 'Chemotherapy', in P. Davies (ed.), *Clinical Tuberculosis* Chapter 14: 243–63 London, Chapman and Hall Medical

Clancy, L. (1998) 'Control of tuberculosis in low-prevalence countries', in P. Davies (ed.), *Clinical Tuberculosis*, Chapter 23: 435–50, London, Chapman and Hall Medical

Crofton, J. (1992) *Clinical tuberculosis*, Basingstoke, Macmillan Press – now Palgrave

Davies, P. (1998) 'Tuberculosis and migration', in P. Davies (ed.), *Clinical Tuberculosis*, Chapter 19:365–82, London, Chapman and Hall Medical

Department of Health and Welsh Office (1996) *The Interdepartmental Working Group on Tuberculosis Guidance and Tuberculosis Control*, London, HMSO

Grange, J., P. Winstanley and P. Davies (1994) 'Clinically significant drug interactions with anti-tuberculosis agents', *Drug Safety*, 11(4) pp. 242–51

Grzybowski, S. (1991) 'Natural history of tuberculosis', *Bulletin of the International Union Against TB and Lung Disease*, 66(4) pp. 193–4

Humphries, M. and W. Lam (1998) 'Non-respiratory tuberculosis', in P. Davies (ed.), *Clinical Tuberculosis*, Chapter 11: 175–204, London, Chapman and Hall Medical

Hunt, L., B. Jordan, S. Irwin and C. Browner (1989) 'Compliance and the patient's perspective: controlling symptoms in everyday life', *Culture, Medicine and Psychiatry*, 13(3) pp. 315–34

Jenkins, J. (1998) 'The microbiology of tuberculosis', in P. Davies (ed.), *Clinical Tuberculosis*, Chapter 5: 69–79, London, Chapman and Hall Medical

JTC (Joint Tuberculosis Committee of the British Thoracic Society) (1994) 'Control and Prevention of Tuberculosis in the United Kingdom: code of practice', *Thorax*, 49(12) pp. 1193–200

JTC (Joint Tuberculosis Committee of the British Thoracic Society) (1998) 'Chemotherapy and Management of Tuberculosis in the United Kingdom: recommendations', *Thorax*, 53(7) pp. 536–48

Kumar, S., J. Innis and C. Skinner (1992) 'Yield from Tuberculosis Contact Screening in Birmingham', *Thorax*, 42(6) pp. 179–82

Leitch, A. (1992) 'Rationalising tuberculosis contact tracing in low-prevalence areas', *Respiratory Medicine*, 86(5) pp. 371–3

Mayho, P. (1998) 'Barrier grief', *Nursing Times*, 95(31) pp. 24–5

Moore-Gillon, J. (1998) 'Tuberculosis and poverty in the developed world', in P. Davies (ed.), *Clinical Tuberculosis*, Chapter 20:383–397, London, Chapman and Hall Medical

Nicas, M. (1995) 'Respiratory protection and the risk of Mycobacterium tuberculosis infection', *American Journal of Industrial Medicine*, 27(3) pp. 317–33

O'Brien, R. (1998) 'Preventive therapy', in P. Davies (ed.), *Clinical Tuberculosis*, Chapter 21:398–416, London, Chapman and Hall Medical

Ormerod, L. (1993) 'Tuberculosis Contact Tracing: Blackburn 1982–90', *Respiratory Medicine*, 87(1) pp. 127–31

Ormerod, L. (1998) 'Respiratory Tuberculosis', in P. Davies (ed.), *Clinical Tuberculosis*, Chapter 10: 155–74, London, Chapman and Hall Medical

Pym, A., D. Churchill, R. Coker and V. Gleissberg (1995) 'Reasons for increased incidence of tuberculosis', *British Medical Journal*, 311(7004) p. 570

Willeke, K. and Y. Qian (1998) 'Tuberculosis control through respirator wear: performance of National Institute for Occupational Safety and Health-regulated respirators', *American Journal of Infection Control*, 26(2) pp. 139–42

Winstanley, P. (1998) 'Clinical pharmacology of antituberculosis drugs', in P. Davies (ed.), *Clinical Tuberculosis*, Chapter 13: 226–42, London, Chapman and Hall Medical

CHAPTER 6

Alteration in Sexuality Pattern: Caring for the HIV Positive Pregnant Woman

JUDITH SUNDERLAND

Patient Profile

Ms F. is a 35 year old woman from Uganda who at the time of meeting the HIV Specialist Midwife had been in the UK for six years. She has a child who was born in Africa in 1988 and still lives there, she no longer has contact with the child's father and although in a stable relationship does not live with her current partner. Ms F. had a vaginal delivery in 1988 in Africa and her wisdom teeth removed under general anaesthetic in 1994. She had hyperemesis during both pregnancies and had been admitted to hospital during the current pregnancy. Ms F.'s mother has hypertension and her grandmother has late onset diabetes.

Risk Factors

There are two categories of risk factors for this client.

1. Risk factors for acquiring HIV infection.
   Ms F. did not identify any risk factors when she underwent the pre-test discussion. However, she is from a country of high prevalence with a sexual history in that country. She also had a dental extraction that following diagnosis she focused on as her source of infection. This remains unproven.
2. The risk factors associated with her diagnosis include:
   Her personal health; the outcome of the pregnancy, and the health of the baby; her 8 year old son's health; and her partner's health.

Chief Complaint

Ms F. presented to the antenatal clinic in the 15th week of her pregnancy. She chose to have an HIV test at the same time as the other blood tests that are recommended at the beginning of pregnancy. She did not identify any risk factors for HIV. The HIV test was positive revealing that she was infected with HIV. Following Ms F.'s diagnosis, her partner had an HIV test, which was negative. The child in Africa remains well, but untested.

Background to Antenatal HIV Testing

It is recommended that all newly pregnant women have an HIV test as part of routine antenatal care (Royal College of Paediatrics and Child Health 1998). This can be performed at the same time as all other routine blood tests. There is much evidence that the risk of transmission of HIV from a pregnant woman to her baby can be greatly reduced by measures taken during the pregnancy, at the time of the delivery, and by the avoidance of breastfeeding. (Connor *et al.* 1994; Dunn *et al.* 1992; European Collaborative Study 1996; Gazzard and Moyle 1998; Mandelbrot *et al.* 1998; Mofenson 1997; Newell 1998; Nicoll *et al.* 2000; Parazzini 1999, Taylor et al 1999; Sunderland 2000). A pregnant woman can only have access to these interventions if her HIV status is known, either prior to or during the pregnancy.

The prevalence of HIV in pregnant women in Newham is consistently the highest in Europe. In 1997, 1:250 babies born at Newham Hospital were born to HIV positive women, (Nicoll *et al.* 1998; PHLS 1998) and the detection rate of women using the maternity service has been low. In 1997 only 1 in 24 women was identified through voluntary named testing. This low identification rate is reflected across London where 75 percent of HIV positive women have remained unidentified (MacDonagh *et al.* 1996a, 1996b; Mercey 1998).

The Royal College of Paediatrics and Child Health Intercollegiate Working Party (1998) recommends that all women have access to HIV testing early and throughout pregnancy, and that in areas of known high prevalence testing should be an integral part of antenatal care. Since the implementation of the Intercollegiate Working Party Guidelines (Royal College of Paediatrics and Child Health 1998) the identification of HIV positive women during pregnancy has improved. Between January 1998 and June 1999, 87 percent of HIV positive women using the maternity services at Newham had been identified; thus enabling treatment for the women and interventions to reduce transmission to the babies.

Definition of the Problem – Pathophysiology

Human immunodeficiency virus (HIV) is a retrovirus. The virus is contained within a lipid membrane or viral envelope and has a viral enzyme reverse transcriptase. Reverse transcriptase enables the virus to make a DNA copy of its RNA genetic material, allowing its integration into the genetic material of the host cell. The virus has an outer glycoprotein gp120 that has a specific affinity to the CD4 cell, which acts as a receptor for the virus. Host cells that contain the CD4 receptor include T4 helper cells, some macrophages and microglial cells in the brain.

The virus becomes a permanent part of the infected persons own cell, and will replicate when the host cell produces more RNA viruses. Following infection with HIV, it was thought that a period of latency occurs. However, there is evidence to suggest that the virus continues to replicate in the lymphatic system in spite of the person remaining asymptomatic. The virus that is now in the nucleus of the host cell will begin to replicate in response to external signals.

In the presence of a new infection the host cell as part of the immune system would normally reproduce itself. However, the cell has been reprogrammed and produces more virus. Once sufficient new viruses have been produced they explode from the host cell through a process known as budding, are released into the blood stream and begin the cycle again by finding other CD4 cells to attack. As a result of the release of the new virus, the host cell membrane will be damaged and the CD4 cell can no longer survive (Pratt 1995).

It is this damage to the immune system caused by the virus that can lead to opportunistic infections and clinical signs and symptoms in an HIV infected person. A diagnosis of AIDS (acquired immune deficiency syndrome) is given when a person infected with HIV develops one of a number of opportunistic infections, as identified by the Communicable Disease Surveillance Centre in Colindale. It is becoming more common for HIV physicians to talk in terms of asymptomatic or symptomatic HIV disease rather than using the term AIDS.

Disease progression is often unpredictable. It is not uncommon for an infected person to be unaware of their HIV status for several years following infection, and also unsure of the source. The risk of transmission during this phase should not be underestimated.

Transmission

Modes of Transmission for HIV include:

Sexual intercourse (anal or vaginal) with an infected person.

Sharing needles with an infected person for intravenous drug use.

Receiving a blood transfusion or other blood products from an infected person.

Vertical transmission (from an HIV infected mother to her baby) either during the pregnancy, at the time of delivery or through breast-feeding.

Transmission of HIV from one person to another is influenced by a number of factors. The virus, that relies upon a host for its survival becomes fragile and easily destroyed once outside the body. For the risk of transmission to increase, the virus needs to be of sufficient quality and quantity and have a direct route of entry into the blood stream of the recipient.

It is difficult to establish degrees of risk for specific activities. Studies have shown conflicting results in different populations, and study samples have not been sizable enough to provide statistical significance. Epidemiological evidence is clear about the activities that pose the greatest risk for HIV transmission (Alcorn 1999).

High Risk:
receptive anal sex;
receptive vaginal sex;
active anal sex;
active vaginal sex;
blood sharing recreational activities;
sharing unsterilised injecting equipment;
being born to an HIV infected mother;
being breast-fed by an HIV infected mother;

Less Risky:
penetrative sex with appropriate barrier (Condom or Femidom). Risk if condom fails;
oral sex;
sharing injecting equipment if inadequately sterilised;
occupational risks in invasive surgical contexts;
laboratory work with super concentrates of HIV.

Very Low Risk:
sharing penetrative sex toys;
sharing razors and tooth brushes;
rimming if blood is present in stool.

Vertical Transmission

The risk of transmission of HIV from an infected mother to her child has global variations. In the developing world where breast-feeding is normal practice, the rate of vertical transmission is about 40 per cent (European Collaborative Study 1992; Peckham and Gibb 1995) and in the developed world 15–20 per cent. (European Collaborative Study 1992). There are certain factors that increase the risk of transmission to the baby. These are:

stage of maternal disease;
high viral load;
low CD4 Count;
seroconversion during pregnancy;
chorioamnionitis;
sexually transmitted infections;
premature delivery;
rupture of membranes of more than four hours prior to delivery;
invasive procedures during labour and delivery;
breastfeeding.
(European Collaborative Study 1996; Landesman *et al.* 1996).

Treatment

Measures to Reduce the Risk of Vertical Transmission

It is important to emphasise that access to interventions to reduce mother to child transmission of HIV will be geographically specific. Globally the majority of babies born with HIV infection will be in areas of the world where resources are scarce and access to health care limited.

Antiretroviral therapy during pregnancy (Gazzard and Moyle 1998; Taylor *et al.* 1999);
treat maternal sexually transmitted infections;
recommend delivery by caesarean section (Mandelbrot *et al.* 1998; Parazzini 1999);
avoid invasive procedures if delivering vaginally, for example: artificial rupture of membranes; fetal scalp electrode; fetal blood sampling; instrumental delivery.
avoid breastfeeding (Dunn *et al.* 1992; Nduati *et al.* 2000).

Planned Outcome of Treatment

For Ms F. to have begun to come to terms with her HIV diagnosis.
To understand the ways she and her partner can reduce the risk of him becoming infected.
To be aware of the way that lifestyle can affect the immune system.
To have commenced an appropriate combination of antiretroviral therapy for herself dependent upon clinical status and surrogate markers.
To have taken the interventions to reduce HIV transmission to the baby.

Domain I – Management of Client Health/Illness Status

Immediate Management

Prior to informing Ms F. of her positive diagnosis, the HIV Specialist Midwife (HIV SM) reflected upon the content of the pre-test discussion with the midwife who performed the test, in order to ascertain any risks identified and to be aware of particular anxieties that the client had. It is important to gain some insight into the client's social background and likely support mechanisms, and the need for language assistance if appropriate. Usual support mechanisms may fail in the presence of HIV due to fear, stigma, ignorance and secrecy (Purnell 1996).

The midwife remembered Ms F. and stated that she was keen to have an HIV test but felt quite confident that the result would be negative. It is not unusual for risk factors for HIV to be overlooked in the antenatal period (Hawken *et al.* 1995) and this has to be born in mind when positive results are being given. The HIV SM wrote to the client to invite her to attend for blood results giving a date and time to come to the antenatal clinic. It is essential that enough time is allocated and an appropriate environment available for giving positive results. Giving positive results on a Friday should be avoided due to the lack of support services at weekends that may be required in the immediate period following diagnosis.

The length of time available should be clarified near the beginning of the session. Based on experience, an hour is an appropriate length of time for this first meeting. It is important that the client has a sense of support and containment at a time when life has been thrown into chaos, and this first meeting will be significant as the beginning of a continuning relationship with the specialist midwife. Having time for the client is a large aspect of the work with HIV positive women, who need both information and support in making decisions within a relatively short period of time. It is important to acknowledge that pregnant women are confined by the time constraints of pregnancy to make certain decisions about disclosure, treatment, mode of delivery and not breastfeeding. Women who are not pregnant and men who are diagnosed with HIV, have many decisions to make, but do not necessarily have the pressure of time constraints that a pregnancy dictates.

Ms F. was very shocked at the news of her positive diagnosis and questioned its accuracy. She said that she felt fine and only had the test to make sure everything was OK. Many women accept an HIV test for this reason, as they want to do everything 'right' during the pregnancy. It is important that the midwife talks with the woman about her likely result prior to taking a test, in order that she is aware that there is a chance that it might be positive even if this seems unlikely.

During this first session it was necessary to achieve a balance between giving information and giving support. The specialist midwife answered Ms F.'s questions, and reassured her that there would be many opportunities throughout the pregnancy for further contact. Ms F.'s immediate concerns were the well being of the pregnancy and the effect that HIV would have on her baby, and the health of her son in Africa. The other main anxiety that Ms F. expressed was how to tell her partner, and would he be infected too. It is common for women to experience difficulty in disclosure to their partners for fear of rejection and blame. This anxiety can contribute to the impact of a positive diagnosis and often lead to the pressure of living with secrets.

Ms F. did tell her partner, who was very supportive. He chose to have a test himself that was negative. Although both Ms F. and her partner were pleased his result was negative, it brought up issues within the relationship that will be discussed in a later section. Ms F. felt able to leave after an hour with the intention of going home and speaking to her partner that evening. The specialist midwife emphasised that both the maternity and the HIV teams have a philosophy of care that incorporates the whole family. It was important for both Ms F. and her partner to be aware that he was welcome to attend all the hospital visits if desired and to feel able to ask for support for himself.

Prior to leaving she was given an appointment for two days time to return to see the HIV physician in conjunction with the HIV specialist midwife. The specialist midwife gave her written information to reinforce what had already been discussed and a contact number should she need to talk in the meantime.

Ongoing Management

An appointment was made for Ms F. to see the HIV physician for an assessment of her health status, and haematological investigations. Advice about appropriate treatment can only be given when viral load and CD4 levels have been measured (Gazzard and Moyle 1998; Taylor *et al.* 1999). It is important to be aware of the anxiety that may surround this first appointment. It may be the first time the woman has been to a sexual health clinic, and she may have fears about being seen in that environment. The first meeting with the HIV physician will reinforce the reality of her diagnosis, as will the literature and written information displayed in the clinic, and the discussion about her own treatment needs based upon the results of her initial blood tests.

Ms F.'s viral load result was 200 copies per ml. and her CD4 count 366. These results indicated that there was no immediate need for her to commence treatment for herself, (Gazzard and Moyle 1998; Taylor *et al.* 1999) but rather to concentrate on the best interventions to reduce transmission to her baby. She was advised that it was good practice to repeat the blood tests in four weeks time in order to get a clear base line from which to work, and that treatment to aid reduction in transmission should commence later in the pregnancy, at around 30 weeks gestation.

The HIV specialist midwife explained to Ms F. that her antenatal care could remain the same as originally planned, but an appointment to see the obstetric consultant would be advised at 34 weeks gestation to discuss and plan mode of delivery. At all stages of the pregnancy, the specialist midwife ensures as far as possible that the woman is having a normal antenatal experience. It is important that the pregnancy is not forgotten in the presence of HIV, and other issues specific to the pregnancy are given the attention they deserve. With permission from Ms F. the community midwife was informed about the HIV in order that conflicting advice could be avoided. For example a midwife may advise a woman to breastfeed, however, in the case of HIV it is strongly recommended that breastfeeding is avoided. If the midwife is aware of the woman's HIV status it is a good opportunity for information and advice about artificial feeding to be given; particularly if she has never bottle-fed before.

As the pregnancy progressed, the specialist midwife referred Ms F. to the family clinic where she saw the HIV paediatrician and the clinical nurse specialist for families and children with HIV. This was another opportunity for her to ask questions about the follow up care her baby would receive and to meet some of the members of the family clinic staff. It was explained to Ms F. that the baby would be seen in the family clinic for 18 months, and be tested for HIV at specific times during that period (Gibb 1998). Antibody testing is not appropriate for babies born to HIV positive mothers, as these babies will acquire the maternal HIV antibody and therefore test positive to an antibody test. It can take up to 18 months for the antibody to be lost from the baby's blood and does not mean that the baby is infected.

To ascertain a baby's HIV status there are a number of tests that can be performed. These are, DNA Polymerase Chain Reaction (PCR), Viral Culture and P24 Antigen (Gibb 1998). If the mother wishes, the baby can have the first test performed before leaving the postnatal ward, and then be seen in the family clinic at one month old for that result and for further testing. The baby should be given zidovudine syrup 2 mg / kg four times a day to commence within four hours of delivery. This should continue for six weeks, and be reviewed in the family clinic. It is advised that babies born to HIV positive mothers should take septrin as a prophylaxis against pneumocystis carinii pneumonia (PCP). This should commence at approximately six weeks when the zidovudine is stopped. Most frequently babies present with PCP at less than 6 months of age. Septrin should continue until it is certain that the baby is negative, but if positive should continue for at least the first year of life.

The outcome of Ms F.'s pregnancy was an elective caesarean section at 38 weeks gestation. She had commenced zidovudine 250 mgs twice daily at 30 weeks gestation, which she found easy to take despite her initial reluctance to start treatment. She had intravenous zidovudine commenced four hours prior to surgery, which continued until the baby was born. She had a baby boy who was given zidovudine syrup 2 mgs/kg four times daily for six weeks. The baby was bottle-fed and has been followed up in the family clinic since birth. It has been confirmed that he is HIV negative.

Domain II – The Midwife–Client Relationship

Immediate Management

The HIV specialist midwife accompanied Ms F. to all her hospital appointments to provide support and act as an advocate when she found it difficult to express her anxieties to other professionals. It was important for Ms F. to know that the specialist midwife was able to contain her anxieties and provide a secure base from which to gain support. Bowlby cited in Purnell (1996) describes the attachment figure as providing a secure base for the affected individual to turn to in times of need. HIV can often threaten usually secure relationships within the family, as diagnosis of HIV for one family member may culminate in the diagnosis of others, who would usually be in a supportive role. It is important that the key professionals are aware of the clients need for reliable and secure relationships as they are supported through diagnosis and decisions about treatment options, disclosure and the future.

Ongoing Management

Ms F. used the time she spent with the specialist midwife to talk through the issues that she found most difficult. She was naturally relieved that her partner was being supportive and that he had tested negative. However she had concerns about their relationship and how they would cope in the future. She said she was afraid of having sex in case he became infected and thought it would be better to stop altogether. Although they were both aware of safer sexual practices and the ways to reduce the risk of transmission, she continued to feel anxious about her ability to contaminate. It is common for specific issues to confront couples where there is serodiscordance (VanDevanter *et al.* 1999) that is one positive and one negative. These include: dealing with the emotional and sexual impact on the relationship; reproductive decisions; planning for the future of children and the surviving partner; disclosure of the HIV infection to family and friends.

Ms F. had anxieties about starting treatment. She said it felt strange to be taking medication when she 'felt fine'. It was suggested to her by the specialist midwife that her reluctance to take medication may mean her HIV becomes a reality, which has to be acknowledged as part of her daily life. Ms F. also was very distressed that it was recommended that she have the baby by caesarean section. Her previous baby was born by vaginal delivery and she had hoped that the same could happen again, with her partner present. She was also worried about how to explain to other people why she had the baby in this way.

The specialist midwife explained that this decision did not need to be made yet, and that she had plenty of time to discuss the procedure with her partner.

It was stressed that it was a recommended mode of delivery, but with the avoidance of certain procedures it was possible that she could have a normal delivery. Ms F. was also very worried about not breastfeeding. She said that it was normal in her culture to breastfeed. If she did not breastfeed, her community would think she was a bad mother, or people would guess that she had HIV.

Anxieties about both not breastfeeding and caesarean delivery often cause a great deal of distress for HIV positive women. Messages about breastfeeding are prominent in antenatal clinics, as it is the recommended mode of feeding for most babies. This, and the associated cultural issues, can contribute to the distress some women experience around decisions made in the presence of HIV. Ms F.'s eventual decision to have a caesarean and not breastfeed was made in good time for the necessary arrangements to be made.

In the majority of cases women accept the interventions that are recommended to reduce transmission, and with support bottle-feed their babies successfully. The specialist midwife ensured that Ms F. was in receipt of all the financial benefits to which she was entitled in order that she was able to purchase the necessary equipment and milk powder. It is important for women who are asylum seekers to be aware of the benefits of referral to social services in order for financial assistance to be arranged where appropriate for the purchase of feeding equipment.

During these sessions Ms F. talked about her fear of becoming ill due to contamination from other people. She described returning from the hairdressers and washing her hair four times before she felt clean. In the same way she talked of her obsessive need to clean the bath both before and after using it. She said that this need to clean was exhausting and debilitating in itself but it was hard to stop. The specialist midwife wondered whether she may be attempting to wash away the virus, and although Ms F. laughed at this idea the obsessive washing gradually stopped over the next weeks. It is easy to take at face value what the client is saying, but it can be helpful to think about the underlying anxieties and what is not being said by the client. It may be the professional's ability to put something in to words on behalf of the client that allows anxieties to be allayed. Working with countertransference feelings can also provide some insight into the client's feelings and what is not being expressed in words. Countertransference feelings are the feelings evoked in the professional by the client. These feelings are communicated at an unconscious level and can manifest in the professional as feelings of fear, anxiety, anger or powerlessness. It is important for the professional to be able to recognize where these feelings belong, in order to help the client make sense of what is happening (O'Kelly 1997).

This relationship can only develop if the woman feels able to trust the professionals and believes that her confidentiality is being maintained. It is important for the specialist midwife to maintain professional boundaries and to encourage the woman to develop other support networks away from the hospital. Fear of loss of confidentiality can lead to secrecy and isolation, but many women feel able to join groups where they have the opportunity to talk with other women with similar experiences.

On the day of admission prior to delivery the specialist midwife visited Ms F. on the ward to answer any last minute questions. It was important for Ms F. at this time to see someone familiar, and her anxieties about confidentiality could be addressed with the staff. She had been particularly anxious that the baby should not be given medication in front of any visitors except her partner, and that the prescription chart should not be left in her room. This was a good opportunity for the specialist midwife to introduce Ms F. and her partner to the midwives who would be caring for her, and to highlight these anxieties.

Domain III – The Teaching Coaching Function

Immediate Management

It was important for the specialist midwife to ensure that Ms F. had a good understanding of her medical condition. There is often confusion about the difference between HIV and AIDS, which is reinforced by the media which consistently fails to make a distinction between the two. Ms F. understood that HIV is the virus that leads to AIDS and her main concern was when would she become sick.

Ms F. also needed information about risk reduction to her partner and her social contacts. She knew about condom use, but was scared about playing with and cuddling her friend's child. The specialist midwife explained that there was no risk from social contact and emphasized the importance of washing and covering any cuts or abrasions she may sustain. The specialist midwife explained to Ms F. the blood tests that would be required before deciding on a treatment plan. It was explained in terms of the viral load measuring the amount of HIV in her blood stream, and the CD4 count as a way of measuring the extent of damage to the immune system. These two blood tests become a familiar aspect of life for people with HIV, so it is important that explanations are clear and simple.

Ongoing Management

While on the postnatal ward the midwives administered the zidovudine syrup to the baby. The specialist midwife ensured that the staff had shown Ms F. how to do this herself, as the baby would require medication for a further five weeks after discharge. In the same way it was necessary to ensure that Ms F. felt confident in preparing bottle feeds, particularly as she had breast-fed her first baby. The specialist midwife reminded the staff who were caring for Ms F. that, although this was her second baby, she would need support and assumptions should not be made about her needs. Staff were also reminded that Ms F. was not bottle feeding out of choice but rather because it had been recommended as better for her baby. It is an easy assumption to make that a woman having her second baby will need less help. However, the needs of newly diagnosed HIV positive mothers should not be underestimated, regardless of how many babies they have already had.

Prior to discharge the specialist midwife had a discussion with Ms F. about her future contraception. Contraceptive advice and information is an important aspect of postnatal management of all women. Discussions about condom use as a risk reduction strategy between serodiscordant couples is essential. However specific contraceptive needs should not be overlooked. It is good practice to liaise with family planning colleagues in order that the most appropriate advice can be given.

The HIV specialist midwife is responsible for the HIV training needs of maternity staff within Newham Healthcare Trust. A two-day training course on a monthly basis provides midwives with the skills to perform antenatal pre-test discussion and also prepares midwives to care for known positive women through pregnancy, delivery and the postnatal period. These study days are co-facilitated by the specialist midwife and a sexual health trainer from East London and the City Health Authority.

Other training involves work with student midwives, medical staff, community groups and midwifery refresher courses. The training requirements around antenatal HIV testing are increasing across London and nationally due to the Intercollegiate Guidelines (Royal College of Paediatrics and Child Health 1998) which have required maternity units to consider the implementation of new policies. There is an increasing opportunity for HIV specialist midwives to provide training for other trusts, as they develop antenatal HIV testing policies.

Domain IV – Professional Role

Immediate Management

As outlined by Trust policy the HIV specialist midwife should be clear about her role and responsibilities. These include:

- Making appropriate referrals as already discussed. Making the necessary arrangements for the caesarean section, including ensuring that the appropriate medication is prescribed and available and the ward staff are aware of the plan of care.
- To ensure that the appropriate staff are aware of the procedure for HIV testing the baby and that follow up care is arranged. A smooth handover to the community staff is essential in providing supportive continuity of care.
- To offer support and information to other professionals involved in the care of the client.
- To have fortnightly consultations to reflect upon practice and specific issues that may emerge with clients. Reflecting on countertransference feelings

evoked by the client is a helpful tool to gain insight into what may be going on for the client that is not being verbalised.
- Maintain links with other HIV specialist midwives through the HIV Maternity Forum, for updating and networking.
- To be actively involved in writing policies that impact on client care, with due regard for evidenced based practice and medical research.

As part of their professional role the HIV specialist midwife should be aware of any articles or reports in the media that give the public information about pregnancy, HIV and antenatal testing. This subject evokes strong feelings among the communities they care for, and it is essential that media information is correct and not misleading. A multi-disciplinary response has occasionally been necessary to clarify facts or to allay anxieties about antenatal HIV testing policies. These responses have always been with the full knowledge and support of the Trust.

Domain V – Managing and Negotiating Health Care Delivery Systems

The specialist midwife ensured that Ms F.'s antenatal care was appropriate to her obstetric needs and not dominated by HIV. It was important to achieve a balance between the need for specialist input and routine care, and as an extension of this to safeguard against undermining or deskilling midwives. This was achieved by acting in a supportive capacity and being clear about roles and boundaries as outlined in trust policies, protocols and guidelines.

Due to the number of professionals involved in the care of Ms F., the specialist midwife ensured that nothing was either duplicated or missed, and this required effective communication and negotiation.

Domain VI – Monitoring and Ensuring the Quality of Health Care Practice

The specialist midwife keeps written records of each contact with all clients, which are kept in the HIV medical notes in the HIV clinic following delivery and at handover to the community staff. The HIV midwife provides the opportunity for staff to discuss individual cases at a monthly support meeting. The aim of this meeting is to give staff the opportunity and space to express anxieties, clarify issues and reflect upon care. Managing confidentiality in the clinical environment can cause anxiety for both staff and clients, particularly when partners and family are not aware of the woman's status.

The HIV midwife is also responsible for monitoring specific aspects of the antenatal HIV testing service. These include:

the uptake of antenatal HIV testing on a monthly basis;
the number of women diagnosed through antenatal HIV testing;
the number of HIV positive women using the maternity service;
the number of midwives trained including new staff within three months of commencing employment;
the HIV results of babies born to HIV positive women;

In addition to this record a confidential log is maintained containing information about individual women's blood results, medication, mode of delivery and outcomes. This data is used as the basis for audit and monitoring workload.

Uptake of antenatal HIV testing is influenced by certain variables. Individual midwives will test a varying number of women, regardless of attending the same training and working within the same policies and guidelines. This is a phenomenon that has been described in the literature (Meadows *et al.* 1990; Simpson *et al.* 1998) and is clearly demonstrated in practice. Cultural and language barriers can impact upon a woman's understanding of the services being offered (Sherr *et al.* 1999) and accurate risk assessment by some women is poor (Hawken *et al.* 1995). As a consequence some women fail to recognize HIV as an issue for them and decline testing (Sunderland 2000). The HIV specialist midwife is responsible for ensuring that the system allows the majority of women to take an HIV test and feel supported through the process. The women who chose not to take the test should be doing so out of choice and not because the system has failed them.

References

Alcorn, K. (1999) *HIV Transmission, National AIDS Manual*, London, NAM Publications

Connor, E., R. Sperling and R. Gelber (1994) 'Reduction of Maternal–Infant Transmission of Human Immunodeficiency Virus Type 1 With Zidovudine Treatment', *New England Journal of Medicine*, 331(18) pp. 1173–80

Department of Health (1996) *Guidelines for Offering Named HIV Antibody Testing to Women Receiving Antenatal Care*, London, HMSO

Dunn, D., M. Newell, A. Ades and C. Peckham (1992) 'Risk of Human Immunodeficiency Virus Type–1 Transmission Through Breast Feeding', *Lancet*, 340(8827) pp. 585–8

European Collaborative Study (1992) 'Risk Factors for Mother to Child Transmission of HIV1', *Lancet*, 339(8800) pp. 1007–12

European Collaborative Study (1996) 'Vertical Transmission of HIV1: Maternal Immune Status and Obstetric Factors', *AIDS*, 10(14) pp. 1675–81

Gazzard, B. and G. Moyle (1998) 'Revision of the British HIV Association Guidelines for Anti-Retroviral Treatment of HIV Sero Positive Individuals', *Lancet*, 352(9124) pp. 314–16

Gibb, D. (1998) *Guidelines for the Management of Children with HIV Infection*, 3 edn, London, Avert

Hawken, J., T. Chard, K. Costeloe, D. Jeffries and C. Hudson (1995) 'Risk Factors for HIV Infection Overlooked in Routine Antenatal Care', *Journal of the Royal Society of Medicine*, 88(11) pp. 634–646

Landesman, S., L. Kalish, D. Burns, H. Minkoff, H. Fox, C. Zorilla, P. Garcia, M. Fowler, L. Mofenson and R. Tuomala (1996) 'Obstetrical Factors and the Transmission of HIV from Mother to Child', *New England Journal of Medicine*, 334(25) pp. 1617–23

MacDonagh, S., J. Masters, B. Helps, P. Tookey, A. Ades and D. Gibb (1996a) 'Descriptive Survey of Antenatal Testing in London: Policy, Uptake and Detection', *British Medical Journal*, 313(7056) pp. 532–3

MacDonagh, S., J. Masters, B. Helps, P. Tookey and D. Gibb (1996b) 'Why are Antenatal HIV Testing Policies in London Failing?' *British Journal of Midwifery*, 4,(9) pp. 466–70

Mandelbrot, L., J. Le Chenadec, A. Berrebi, A. Bongain and J. Benifla (1998) 'Perinatal HIV-1 Transmission: interaction between Zidovudine prophylaxis and mode of delivery in the French Perinatal Cohort', *JAMA*, 280(1) pp. 55–60

Meadows, J., S. Jenkins, J. Catalan and B. Gazzard (1990) 'Voluntary HIV Testing in the Antenatal Clinic: Differing Uptake Rates for Individual Counselling Midwives', *AIDS Care*, 2(3) pp. 229–33

Mercey, D. (1998) 'Antenatal HIV Testing has been done badly in Britain and needs to improve', *British Medical Journal*, 316(7127) pp. 241–2

Mofenson, L. (1997) 'Efficacy of Zidovudine in Reducing Perinatal HIV-1 Transmission in HIV-1 Infected Women with Advanced Disease', abstract in Proceedings of the 37th Interscience Conference on Anti-Retroviral Agents and Chemo Therapy, Toronto, Canada

Nduati, R., D. Mbori-Ngacha, B. Richardson, J. Overgaugh, A. Mwatha, J. Ndinya-Achola, J. Bwayo, F. Onyango, J. Hughes and J. Kreiss (2000) 'Effect of breastfeeding and formula feeding on transmission of HIV-1: a randomised clinical trial', *JAMA*, 283(9) pp. 1167–74

Newell, M. (1998) 'Mechanisms and Timing of Mother to Child Transmission of HIV-1', *AIDS*, 12(8) pp. 831–7

Nicoll, A., C. McGarrigle, A. Brady, A. Adgs and P. Tookey (1998) 'Epidemiology and Detection of HIV-1 Among Pregnant Women in the United Kingdom: Results from national surveillance 1988–1996', *British Medical Journal*, 316(7127) pp. 253–9

Nicoll, A., M. Newell, C. Peckham, C. Luo and F. Savage (2000) 'Infant Feeding and HIV-1 Infection–Year 2000 (Review)', *AIDS 14* (Supplement 3) pp. 557–74

O'Kelly, G. (1997) 'Countertransference in the Nurse Patient Relationship: A Review of the Literature', *Journal of Advanced Nursing*, 28(2) pp. 391–7

Parazzini, F. (1999) 'For the European Mode of Delivery Collaboration, Elective Caesarean Section Versus Vaginal delivery in Prevention of Vertical HIV-1 Transmission: A Randomised Controlled Trial', *Lancet*, 353(9158) pp. 1035–9

Peckham, C. and D. Gibb (1995) 'Mother to Child Transmission of HIV-1', *New England Journal of Medicine*, 333(5) pp. 298–302

Pratt, R. (1995) *AIDS: A Strategy for Nursing Care*, 4th edn, London, Edward Arnold

Public Health Laboratory Service (1998) *Unlinked Anonymous HIV Prevalence Monitoring Programme: England and Wales*, Survey of Antenatal Attenders, London, Colindale

Purnell, C. (1996) 'An Attachment Based Approach to Working with Clients Affected by HIV and AIDS', *British Journal of Psychotherapy*, 12(4) pp. 521–31

Royal College of Paediatrics and Child Health (1998) *Intercollegiate Working Party for Enhancing Voluntary Confidential HIV Testing in Pregnancy*, London, Royal College of Paediatrics and Child Health, April

Sherr, L., A. Bergonstrom, E. Bell, E. McCann and C. Hudson (1999) 'Antenatal HIV Screening in Ethnic Minority Women', *Health Trends* 1998/9, 30(4) pp. 115–19

Simpson, W., F. Johnstone, F. Boyd, G. Hart, D. Goldberg and R. Prescott (1998) 'Uptake and Acceptability of Antenatal HIV Testing: Randomised Controlled Trial of Different Methods of Offering the Test', *British Medical Journal*, 316(7127) pp. 262–7

Sunderland, J. (2000) 'Increasing Uptake of Antenatal HIV Testing in Newham Healthcare NHS Trust: The Implementation of a New Approach to Antenatal Testing', *MIDRS Midwifery Digest* 10,(1) pp. 31–4

Taylor, G., H. Lyall, D. Mercey, R. Smith, T. Chester, M. Newell and G. Tudor-Williams (1999) 'British HIV Association Guidelines for Prescribing Anti Retroviral Therapy in Pregnancy', *Sexually Transmitted Infections*, 75(2) pp. 90–7

VanDevanter, N., A. Stuart-Thacker, G. Bass and M. Arnold (1999) 'Heterosexual Couples Confronting the Challenges of HIV Infection', *AIDS Care*, 11(2) pp. 181–93

CHAPTER 7

Alteration in Endocrine Function: Caring for the Woman in Obstetric Crisis

JOANNE HUTCHINSON

Patient Profile

Mrs G. is a 22 year old Asian housewife and mother of two girls: ages one year and nine months, respectively. She is a practicing Muslim. Her first language is Urdu but she speaks English quite well. Having emigrated from Pakistan two years ago, her social support includes her husband and his immediate and extended family.

Risk Factors

Medically, Mrs G.'s condition was satisfactory, but she has a strong family history of diabetes and hypertension. Her obstetric history was poor; in addition to having a consanguineous marriage and being overweight, Mrs G. had a previous miscarriage and stillbirth at 13 and 38 weeks, respectively.

Chief Complaint

In view of the risk factors with which Mrs G. presented, and based on the evidence which supports screening for similar clients, she was offered an Oral Glucose Tolerance Test (OGTT) at 16 and 28 weeks gestation according to the local district wide guidelines. Mrs G. was diagnosed as having Gestational diabetes mellitus (GDM) based on the 16 weeks result. Her fasting blood glucose was high: 10.1 mmol/L (1 mmol = 18 mg/dl); the test was terminated and diagnosis was made using the local assessment criteria (see Table 7.1). Consequently, Mrs G. was monitored closely in the joint obstetric/medical diabetic clinic at Newham Healthcare Trust.

Table 7.1 Gestational Diabetes Mellitus: Local Assessment Criteria

Normal	*Gestational Diabetes Mellitus*
Blood Glucose (mmol/L) 0 min – < 6.0 and 120 min – < 7.8	Blood Glucose (mmol/L) > 6.0 or > 7.8

Source: World Health Organisation Standards (2000) June

Table 7.2 Risk Factors for Gestational Diabetes

Family history	Previous gestational diabetes
Poor obstetric history	Previous large baby (>4 kg)
History of high blood pressure	Pre-eclampsia
Polyhydramnios	> age 40 and no children within 5yrs

Other Complaints

Mrs G. was very anxious on discovering that she had GDM. She appeared to have experienced a loss of her normal state and patterned the grief process described by Kubler-Ross (1984). Anxieties were raised around her fear of needles and having to receive insulin therapy. She also feared that her baby would die as a result of the insulin. Being diagnosed as having GDM, and having had two girls previously, Mrs G. feared that her condition and its management would reduce the chance of her having a boy child – a necessity for status and acceptance within her family (Henley 1979; Sen 1989). Nevertheless, having an addition to her family, irrespective of the baby's sex was worthwhile, considering her previous obstetric history and the need for her to increase her family size to prove her status and enhance self-worth.

Remaining diabetic after pregnancy was another concern. Mrs G. also experienced difficulties adjusting from a high fat and sugar diet to that of a diabetic diet. Although conventional therapy was eventually accepted in order to manage her diagnosis adequately, Mrs G. also received complementary therapy from a traditional healer. Despite having difficulties coming to terms with the fact that she had GDM, Mrs G. became more accepting of her condition and was able to manage her condition with great confidence.

Definition of the Problem – Pathophysiology

Prevalence/Incidence

The prevalence and incidence of GDM varies between populations. In the United Kingdom and most of Europe, the overall reported incidence is between 1 and 2 per cent (Donhorst *et al.* 1992; Pickup and Williams 1991). A large multi-ethnic study conducted by Donhorst *et al.* (1992) has shown a higher incidence of GDM in the non-indigenous population with a relative risk of 3.1 per cent for blacks, 7.6 per cent for South East Asians and 11.3 per cent for women from the Indian subcontinent. A retrospective study by Akter *et al.* (1996) among Pakistani women living in Karachi showed an incidence of 3.3 per cent.

The local clientele comprises highly of the non-indigenous group. Within this clientele, the prevalence of GDM remains unknown, however a recent audit revealed that of 237 antenatal diabetic clinic attendees, 76 per cent had abnormal blood glucose levels. Thirty-three per cent had GDM, while the remainder had Impaired Glucose Tolerance (IGT).

In view of this, and since the childbearing age appears to be younger for local first-time mothers, it may be concluded that the prevalence of GDM will continue to proliferate. Another confounding factor is the fact that Type II diabetes mellitus (DM) (formerly non-insulin dependent diabetes mellitus – NIDDM) is known to have generic components, and is common among the non-indigenous population (Hawthorne *et al.* 1993).

In view of the incidence and prevalence of GDM, the need for universal screening remains crucial, yet controversial (De *et al.* 1997). In response to the local need for the effective management of GDM and diabetes in general, the Shrewsbury Road Diabetic Centre was established. The Diabetic Midwife's (DM) post was later created to care primarily for pregnant women with abnormal blood glucose levels.

Physiology

Gestational diabetes mellitus is best described as glucose intolerance that first presents during pregnancy (Jarrett 1993; Pickup and Williams 1991). GDM develops at any time, but most commonly during the second and third trimester (Pickup and Williams 1991). Pregnancy has been described as *diabetogenic* (Kyne-Grzebalski *et al.* 1994). The impact of GDM on pregnancy is similar to that of overt diabetics (Pickup and Williams 1991) and by definition includes a small number of women with previously unrecognised diabetes or IST (Donhorst *et al.* 1992). Progesterone, oestrogen, lactogen, cortisol and human placental levels increase during pregnancy and combined these hormones determine the level of blood glucose. In most women the pancreas compensates by progressively secreting insulin to meet the required level which results in the blood glucose level remaining fairly constant. GDM develops if the pancreas is unable to meet this physiological demand.

Morbidity/Mortality

The risks of GDM on the pregnancy, although generally fewer and less severe, are similar to that of known diabetics (Pickup and Williams, 1991). Despite the improved management of GDM in specialist centres by specialist teams, and with the advent of self-blood glucose monitoring, maternal and fetal morbidity and mortality among GDMs remain higher than that of the non-GDM population (Akter *et al.* 1996). The following evidence emphasises the importance of early detection and aggressive management of GDM.

Effects on the fetus

The most commonly reported complication of GDM is macrosomia and its associated problems. Fetal growth accelerates, especially during the third trimester, and birth weights can exceed the 97th centile (Jarrett 1997; Maresh *et al.* 1989; O'Sullivan *et al.* 1973a; Watkins, 1998). One study suggested that if GDM remains untreated, 4 per cent of women compared with 2 per cent of the non-GDM population would deliver infants weighing 4500 gms or more (Ales and Sanitini 1989). An agreed consensus is yet to be reached around the parameters of macrosomia (Jarrett 1997). Nevertheless, a large baby is more at risk of shoulder dystocia and birth trauma. The incidence of the rate of stillbirth us also increased (Pickup and Williams 1991) in this population.

Effects on the neonate

The efficacy of treatment during pregnancy tends to determine neonatal well-being. Hypoglycaemia, respiratory distress syndrome, jaundice and all other complications affecting babies of known diabetics, may occur (Hawthorne *et al.* 1993; James *et al.* 1984; Pickup and Williams 1991).

Effects on the child

Recent studies have highlighted the effects of the intrauterine environment on future adult chronic diseases (Abraha *et al.* 1999; Barker and Martyn 1992; Fraser and Bruce 1999). A longitudinal study carried out within the Puma Indian population showed that children of diabetic mothers were at greater risk of developing diabetes and childhood obesity than other siblings born to these mothers before they were diagnosed as diabetics (Pettitt *et al.* 1988). It remains uncertain as to whether children born to GDM mothers are affected. Further research needs to be undertaken in this area.

A theory is emerging that indicates maternal carbohydrate metabolism may also influence fetal insulin secretion and function. Infants born to diabetic mothers have greater insulin resistance and are more likely to have glucose intolerance during puberty (Silverman *et al.* 1995).

Effects on the mother

The risk to the mother may be described as comparatively small, but is an essential indicator for health promotion and health education. The mother is exposed to the trauma of giving birth to a large baby. Hence, the increase in caesarean section deliveries among women with GDM (Fraser and Bruce 1999; Jarrett 1993). The detection of GDM identifies women at risk of developing future permanent diabetes (Bushard *et al.* 1987), of which NIDDM is more common (Akter *et al.* 1996; Dornhorst *et al.* 1990; O'Sullivan 1982). A metabolic disturbance may exist in the mother and be active for as long as 20 years before diabetes is diagnosed. The rate of progression depends predominantly on age, parity, family history, ethnicity and the degree of glucose intolerance and weight, during and after pregnancy (Metzger *et al.* 1993). For Asians, about 40 per cent of women with GDM will develop diabetes within six years, while 70 per cent will develop impaired glucose intolerance (IGT) (Kjos *et al.* 1995). The rate of progression to diabetes is marginally lower among Europeans, that is, 20–40 per cent within 20 years (Henry *et al.* 1993).

Screening

Women with GDM tend to remain asymptomatic, except for experiencing rapid fetal growth during the latter part of their pregnancy. In view of this, and the fact that there is a global epidemic of Type II DM, especially among the non-indigenous population (Simmons *et al.* 1989), best practice mandates that antenatal clinics should have the necessary provision for early detection and subsequent appropriate management (Jornsay *et al.* 1997). This must be coupled with radical preventative measures (Buchanan, 1995; Manson *et al.* 1991) if morbidity and mortality associated to GDM are to be reduced.

Detection of GDM can be made from either a random blood glucose or an OGTT which is the more common and accurate option. The exact glucose load to perform an OGTT, and the diagnostic level at which treatment for GDM is required, remains controversial. Hence, the need for one test and one diagnostic criterion is recognized (Khandelwal *et al.* 1999; Nelson- Piercy and Gale 1993).

The modified OGTT test remains the gold standard. This involves a two-hour OGTT with a 75 g glucose load – a measure used during and outside pregnancy. It is postulated that this test has 95 per cent sensitivity and approximately 85 per cent specificity for detecting GDM between 20 and 28 weeks gestation. A first trimester test (before 20 weeks gestation) is highly recommended since women in the High Risk category (Table 7.2) are more likely to develop GDM before the second trimester (O'Sullivan *et al.* 1973b; Weeks *et al.* 1994; Pickup and Williams, 1991).

Treatment

Management of GDM can be either diet control alone or diet control with insulin therapy, following self-blood glucose monitoring (Buchanan 1995; Akter *et al.* 1996)

The role of the Diabetic Midwife (DM), together with other members of the diabetic team, is to ensure that clients are educated through an appropriate teaching strategy about the changes that occur, while providing adequate and sensitive support to enable clients to have a pregnancy outcome similar to that of the non-diabetic mother.

Domain I – Management of Client Health/Illness Status

Immediate Management

The philosophy of care when caring for high risk women should be one that promotes the elements embedded within the notion of clinical governance. Otherwise, women, rightfully so, may challenge health professionals to produce the evidence underpinning their practice. Failure to respond adequately may suggest that health professionals are negligent in their practice.

The diagnosis of GDM and the management of clients with this condition can be a very complex and challenging experience for many. This complexity was highlighted when gestational diabetes and its management was described as being controversial by Jarrett (1997). It was therefore imperative to expedite immediate transfer of Mrs G.'s care to the joint obstetric/medical diabetic clinic, with a view to providing the best care possible for her and her baby.

With the use of the best evidence available, the goal was to strive for a positive outcome for mother and baby. To achieve this, Mrs G. had to be assessed within the context of her family, friends, society and environment. Based on this understanding, an adequate plan of care was developed (Aggleton and Chalmers 1989).

The term *Asian* hides a diversity of attributes such as language, religion, place of origin and social class between the different groups. Even within these groups are subgroups, thus highlighting the need for individualised care. Hence, Asian clients should be treated as individuals within their cultural context.

On her first visit to the Diabetic Clinic, Mrs G. was seen by a Diabetic Nurse Specialist (DNS), a dietitian and the DM – all of whom explained the results of the OGTT, and the risk factors associated with GDM. The requirements to manage this condition successfully were also discussed. It was also the prime duty of the DM to orientate Mrs G. to the clinic and to reassure her that as the only midwife attached to the clinic, the DM was available to address any concerns that she might have pertaining to the pregnancy. On subsequent visits, Mrs G. was also cared for by the consultant obstetrician and consultant diabetologist from whom she received joint consultative care.

The DNS taught self-monitoring of blood glucose levels – an exercise which Mrs G. had to carryout twice daily until delivery. The aim was for blood glucose levels to be within the ranges of 4–6 mmol/L pre-prandial and < 7 mmol/L post-prandial. The benefits of self-monitoring relative to the improvement and stabilisation of blood glucose levels, and ultimately, the improvement in maternal and fetal outcome, are well documented (Hounsome 1998). Blood was also taken for baseline fructosamine levels. This gives a more accurate reading of the blood glucose series over a maximum period of three weeks when compared to HA1c levels which covers a longer period of time (Parfitt *et al.* 1993). A dietary assessment by the dietitian revealed the need for modification in Mrs G.'s dietary lifestyle. Her very high fat and sugar intake was reflective of a typical Asian diet (Hawthorne *et al.* 1993).

Ongoing Management

On average, Mrs G. was reviewed fortnightly in the Diabetic Clinic although she was seen weekly in the embryonic stage. Monthly scans followed by fortnightly ones, were arranged to monitor fetal well-being, particularly for macrosomia (Saunders and James 1985). After a week of diet therapy and self-monitoring, an assessment was made to determine whether a change in management was necessary. Mrs G. had not monitored her blood glucose and was therefore unable to produce any record of her blood glucose levels for that week. That aspect of care required further teaching by the DM, which proved effective. Her blood glucose level when checked on that visit was 10.7 mmol/L, three hours post-prandial. This indicated that insulin therapy was necessary. This form of treatment was initially declined due to fear of needles and fear that such treatment would have harmed the baby. It was later accepted after reassurance and support was given. The fear of self-administration of insulin was overcome after the decision was made that Mrs G.'s sister-in-law would administer the insulin after being taught to do so. The insulin requirement and its frequency varied progressively during her pregnancy. Mrs G. was initially prescribed 12 units of mixtard in the morning and 8 units in the evening.

During the first month following the diagnosis, Mrs G.'s blood glucose levels fluctuated between the ranges of 4.6 and 11.3mmols. Lack of stabilisation of blood glucose levels was linked to the difficulties of adhering to a diabetic diet due to cultural and social reasons. Lack of compliance was also manifest in the occasional glycosuria and high fructosamine levels. With extra help and support, while paying particular attention to the reasons explained for non-compliance, Mrs G.'s blood glucose levels were within the normal ranges at 29 weeks gestation, and remained that way until delivery.

Between 32 and 34 weeks gestation Mrs G. went to Pakistan for a short break to spend time with her family. Unlike many Pakistani women – who stop conventional treatment, as they believe that temperature and sweating reduce blood sugar levels (Hawthorne *et al.* 1993) – Mrs G. continued the combined use of complementary (herbal) and conventional treatment and successfully managed her condition. Fetal size remained normal and plans were made for a normal vaginal delivery following induction of labour at 38 weeks gestation.

At 37 weeks gestation, Mrs G. went into spontaneous labour and gave birth to a baby boy weighing 3288 gms. Management during labour involved the simultaneous use of intravenous fluid 5–10 dextrose and the use of a *sliding scale* (see Table 7.3) at the onset of labour, during which time hourly blood glucose levels were checked while Mrs G. remained nil by mouth. A sliding scale consisting of 50 units of actrapid insulin in 50mls of normal saline was commenced and adjusted according to the hourly readings. Immediately after delivery all insulin therapy was ceased and blood glucose levels were monitored every six hours for 24 hours.

The baby's blood glucose level immediately post delivery was 2.3 mmols. By keeping the baby warm and with early feeds, the baby's blood glucose level satisfactorily increased and admission into the neighbouring Special Care Baby

Table 7.3 Sliding Scale

Blood Monitoring Reading Units/Hour (mmol/L)		*Actrapid (ml/hr)*
<4 mmol/L	–	0.5 ml/hr
4.1–7 mmol/L	–	1 ml/hr
7.1–9 mmol/L	–	1.5 ml/hr
9.1–11 mmol/L	–	2 ml/hr
11.1–14 mmol/L	–	3 ml/hr
14.1–17 mmol/L	–	4 ml/hr
> 17 mmol/L Doctor		6 + Call

(50 units Actrapid in 50 ml normal saline –1 unit = 1 ml)

Unit was not necessary. Assessment of blood glucose levels continued prior to three-hourly feeds for 24 hours.

Mrs G.'s blood glucose level immediately following delivery was 4.7 mmols. Subsequent readings during the first 24 hour period, according to local policy, were all satisfactory. Consequently, no further testing and insulin therapy was required. Nevertheless, a three months postnatal OGTT appointment was arranged. The result of this test determines whether or not clients proceed to be classified as *true diabetics.* The DM had to explicitly communicate this information to both Mrs G. and the midwives responsible for her care, since the result of the test was crucial in determining future plans of care, especially during subsequent pregnancies (Pickup and Williams, 1991).

For Mrs G., the result of that test was IGT, suggesting that her blood glucose level was higher than normal, but not high enough to diagnose diabetes mellitus. Hence, Mrs G. was advised to continue to adhere to a diabetic diet and to loose weight. Her GP was informed of the results and it was recommended that she be reviewed on an annual basis with random blood glucose measurements. Any additional support that the GP needs can be obtained from the hospital staff but primarily from the specialist centre at Shrewsbury Road.

Domain II – The Nurse–Client Relationship

Immediate Management

The elicitation of Mrs G.'s abnormally high blood glucose level from the 16 weeks OGTT result, by local criteria (Table 7.1), necessitated prompt referral to the antenatal diabetic clinic, where she was closely monitored. At present, recent evidence suggests that clinics should have arrangements in place for early detection and subsequent management of clients like Mrs G.

Having received the chemical pathology report, the role of the DM was to contact Mrs G. immediately and explain the findings of the report and answer any questions that she had. Reassurance, through explanation based on research, was given. Discussion around the likelihood that her condition may be temporary was like music to Mrs G.'s ears. In view of the benefits derived from acknowledging *honesty as a management virtue* (Phillips *et al.* 1994) and enabling clients to make informed decisions through the provision of adequate information (Buchanan 1995), it was imperative to mention that research evidence suggests that some women with GDM still remain diabetic following delivery (Donhorst and Rossi 1998; O'Sullivan 1984).

Bearing in mind the turmoil experienced during pregnancy (Niven 1992), especially women whose pregnancies are complicated with GDM (Jarrett, 1997), sensitivity was displayed when breaking the news. Good communication with the mother and her partner/relatives engenders trust and subsequently builds good working relationships. The quality of midwifery care also improves. This encourages the mother to accept midwifery advice especially if complications arise necessitating departure from a previously agreed plan of care (Newton 1991).

The initial telephone conversation included basic dietary advice and mention was made that an in-depth assessment would be made of her situation on her first visit to the antenatal diabetic clinic. An appointment was given for the next clinic session. Contact numbers were also given to Mrs G. should she need to discuss any concerns prior to her clinic appointment. Clients need time to express themselves and this is not always possible in a busy clinic environment. In view of this, the DM gave the reassurance that contact can be made at any time, including seeing her out of clinic hours.

Mrs G., like all first-time attendees to the diabetic clinic, was seen by the DM. The DM took the opportunity on the first visit to orientate Mrs G. to the environment. This was deemed necessary in view of the benefits derived from orientating clients (Matthews 1993); Mrs G. might have been unsure as to what course of action to take when professional help was required. A formal introduction is usually made, after which the structure of the diabetic clinic is described while paying particular attention to outlining each professional's role, inclusive of the DM's within the clinic. Discussions also include the future plan of care.

Part of the DM's role includes ensuring that routine antenatal care was not overlooked. Reassuring clients that the DM can be approached with any problems which may arise is essential, whether such problems are diabetic/pregnancy related or not. This usually sets the scene for the client and tends to form the platform on which a trusting relationship progressively develops between the DM and the client.

Ongoing Management

The DM needed an understanding of Pakistanis' expectations of the health service in order to tailor help sensitively to meet the needs of Mrs G. (Hawthorne and Tomlinson 1999). Like many Asians, Mrs G. followed strict practices as to where men and women should sit in the waiting area, that is, separately. Patience had to be exercised as Mrs G. would go and get her husband from the other side of the room when her name was called for consultation during antenatal clinic visits. Also, the legal bond of marriage and her 'inferior status' as a *woman* do not permit her to control her own situation (Trevelyan 1994). Mrs G. would always seek permission from her husband, whatever the decision to be made. It was, therefore, vital to ensure that decisions made were truly hers and not those of her husband. The guilt women with GDM may feel over taking time-off from their *superwoman* roles of wife and mother in order to care for their own health was addressed with compassion, yet practically, by the DM and other members of the multidisciplinary team.

During later discussions, it was revealed that Mrs G. was also receiving concurrent treatment from a traditional healer. There was no doubt that Mrs G.'s cultural beliefs influenced her decision to seek additional help. This was not a surprise since the reliance of Asians on traditional remedies is well documented. There are two main classes: Ayurvedic medicine is based on plants and herbs and has at its origin Hindu Vedas. The Yuan or Greek medicine is a derivative of powdered medicines from spices, herbs, the barks from certain trees and some heavy metals (Table 7.4) (Aslam *et al.* 1979; Hawthorne 1990; Singh-Bhopal 1986). Mrs G. used a combination of both kinds of medicines and she believed this contributed to the stabilisation of her blood glucose levels. The supplementary ingredients mainly used were the domestic onion, allium sativum (garlic) and momordica charantia (karela), of which the latter is claimed to have much more potent hypoglycaemic properties to treat diabetes (Aslam and Stockley 1979; Chopra *et al.* 1958). Although the above are basic ingredients used in the preparation of curry dishes that formed part of Mrs G.'s daily diet, there is no substantial evidence to support their usage in the management of her condition. Hence further research is needed in these areas.

Mrs G. expressed concerns to the DM that while she would have liked to make a birth plan, because of her situation, she felt that having one was 'a complete waste of time'. Control, information giving, support and decisionmaking were some of the main themes that emerged from a prospective study of women's views of factors contributing to a positive birth experience (Lavender *et al.* 1999). Mindful of this, while recognizing the need for individualised care, Mrs G. was assisted to articulate realistic expectations by formulating an appropriate birth plan which embraced her condition, yet gave her some control over her birth experience.

Table 7.4 Some Herbal and Traditional Remedies used by Diabetic Asians

Momordica charantia	Garlic
Karela	Bitter ground tree
Jamun	
Gula	Banyan tree
Vijesal	
Kakachia	Bitter gall
Methi	Fenugreek
Mushrooms	
Cucumber	
Spinach	
Herbal Tea	
Allium sativum	
Lecithin granules	
Powders and spices, herbs and metals	

As is customary, the DM visited Mrs G. on the postnatal ward. The purpose of that visit was to aid continuity of care and carer, thus providing a familiar face for her to reflect on her experiences. Spending time with clients at that time proves to be beneficial – time is an asset not always available on a busy ward (Enkin *et al.* 1995). Ensuring that clients receive the postnatal OGTT appointment prior to discharge from hospital is also a crucial part of the role of the DM. Clients' care in general (antenatal and throughout) is evaluated on this visit. Positive experiences are shared with the DM in order to maintain high standards of care, while adverse experiences are considered in order to make changes so that an improved service can be provided.

Domain III – The Teaching Coaching Function

Immediate Management

The way women are cared for during pregnancy and childbirth is crucial in laying the foundations of confidence and self-esteem (Niven 1992; Robinson and Thompson 1991). Midwives as *partners in care* should play a significant part in building this confidence by fulfilling their health education and health promotion role (Enkin *et al.* 1995; Raphael-Leff 1991). In view of this, while considering the role of the DM as an all- rounder, she is in a very unique and valued position when caring for GDMs, like Mrs G.

A pilot study conducted to evaluate the care *Asian diabetics attending a British hospital clinic received* revealed that, despite receiving the same education as British diabetics, Asians were less knowledgeable about their condition and its management. Irrelevant advice on diet and customs is believed to be the likely reason, thus contributing to poorer glycaemic control (Hawthorne 1990). Health education must be culturally sensitive both in terms of content and mode of delivery, since an individual's health beliefs are influenced by his/her culture, social background, experience of health and exposure to health promotion behaviour (McAllister and Farquhar 1992).

Although the understanding of these is complex, they play a vital role in determining preventive health behaviour. They act as stimuli to initiate and sustain behaviour as outlined in the health belief model (HBM). The HBM also presents the dimensions of perceived benefits and risks from fashioning particular health behaviours (Rosenstock 1972). Bearing in mind that compliance increases, if a person is well informed (Enkin *et al.* 1995), the benefits and risks of effective self-monitoring and having an appropriate diet, was reiterated to Mrs G., by the DM. Mrs G. remained confused about self-monitoring after being taught self-monitoring on her first clinic visit, by the DNS. This was solely due to the fact that Mrs G. was still shocked about her diagnosis of GDM. Consequently, an appointment was made for her to attend the hospital away from the busy antenatal diabetic clinic environment, to receive reinforcement teaching on how to self-monitor blood glucose levels.

Having considered the above, eliciting and understanding Mrs G.'s own interpretation of her illness was the next crucial stage for assessment to facilitate the teaching/coaching aspect of her care (Benner 1984). Once this was established, plans were systematically made to address her educational needs.

Ongoing Management

Within the Asian culture, anyone who tries to loose weight, as Mrs G. was advised, may be criticised by elderly family members for their *poorly* appearance. Plumpness is indicative of good health and affluence. For example, the amount of ghee on a dish reflects the affluence of the household. It may be argued that the perceived wealth gained from immigrating to Britain may suggest the use of larger amounts of ghee being used among Asians; therefore the greater their fat intake (Hawthorne *et al.* 1993). Ghee also has a sanctity value and is used in religious ceremonies. Being a devout Muslim meant that avoiding ghee was difficult for Mrs G. and required great help and support. This may have contributed to the failed management of Mrs G. on *diet only* therapy.

Apart from giving hospitality, it is imperative for food to be received with good grace. It is considered impolite to refuse food. This can cause embarrassment to clients (Hawthorne *et al.* 1993) as was sometimes experienced by Mrs G. when she visited her mother-in-law daily, while trying to adhere to dietary restrictions. Foods, fall into *hot* and *cold* categories. Cold foods are encouraged during pregnancy, since hot foods such as eggs, dried fruits and lentils are believed to lead to miscarriage (Hawthorne *et al.* 1993). Some of the foods that fall into the *ho*t category are considered healthy and encouraged in the diet especially during pregnancy.

Although the dietitian and the DM have distinctive roles, the latter also needed to be knowledgeable about Asian dietary habits in order to reinforce information previously given. This provides continuous and appropriate care and advice, especially when Mrs G. initially denied her condition. Mrs G. was supported in this aspect of her care. With Mrs G.'s consent, her sister-in-law, who was British born and Westernised, was taught about the need for weight loss, especially when a woman is diagnosed as having GDM. This support was believed to be a contributory factor to Mrs G.'s ultimate compliance with her care.

The local clientele is sometimes described as anything but proactive in relation to their care. This is believed to be due to learnt cultural behaviour. Initially, the stated request from Mrs G. for frequent visits to the clinic implied an external *locus of control.* It was, therefore, vital for efforts to be channelled towards helping her to change her locus of control and take more control of her situation, because only then would she be able to successfully manage her condition. The DM needed to assist in engendering feelings of empowerment, thus enabling Mrs G. to take more control of her situation – a vital element necessary for the successful management of her condition.

Ramadan is an annual period of fasting celebrated by Asian Muslims. Because Mrs G. was pregnant, she could have been exempted from fasting during that period, but she preferred to fast, as missed days must be made up later. With appropriate advice and support on timing of diet and medication (Sulimani *et al.* 1988), Mrs G. fasted without detriment to her or her baby's health.

The role of the DM is also one of support and guidance to clients and their relatives, colleagues, junior doctors and students. The DM also acts as a resource centre for these groups. Formal and informal teaching and information giving form a vital part of the DM's role. Simply being available for reflection in and on practice provides growth and development (Watson 1999).

Domain IV – Professional Role

Immediate Management

Legally, the DM is subject to the same laws that govern midwives in general. That is, the UKCC Professional Code of Conduct (UKCC 1993) and the Midwives Rules (UKCC 1998). Contemporaneous record keeping, advocacy, accountability and responsibility are to name but a few of the DM's duties when caring for women with GDM (Monaghan *et al.* 2000).

The midwife plays a pivotal role in the provision of maternity care throughout the antepartum, intrapartum and postpartum periods. The midwife also provides a high proportion of care for women with pregnancy complications whose care is directly managed by an obstetrician. With this in mind, and being in the exemplary position of a DM, it was her duty to assist Mrs G. to make choices with which she was comfortable, while facilitating appropriate steps towards a more integrated approach to her healthcare management.

Ongoing Management

In view of the complexity of caring for High Risk clients, like those with GDM, the DM needs to critically appraise all aspects of care delivery to ensure the provision of the best possible care to clients. To achieve this, the DM needs to be proactive in gaining relevant knowledge and expertise, and also to be prepared to maximise her role of advocacy (UKCC 1993).

The changing pattern of care has led to the necessity for professionals to be knowledgeable about their work while embracing evidence based practice. Failure to achieve this may result in the DM failing to take appropriate and timely action should any *deviation from the norm* arise, thus neglecting her legal role (UKCC 1993). The DM needs to remember that in exercising her professional accountability, entrusted in her by those laws, she should report to appropriate personnel and authorities any circumstances in which safe and appropriate care for patients/clients cannot be provided (Dimond 1994). In the case of Mrs G., the disclosure of the use of complementary therapy was shared with professionals involved in her care. This was deemed necessary bearing in mind the potency of some traditional medicines.

Domain V – Managing and Negotiating Health Care Delivery Systems

Immediate Management

The Borough of Newham remains one of the more deprived areas in London. Such deprivation is locally and nationally recognised and is believed at times to contribute to substandard care. Negotiating for changes in management of care delivery, can sometimes be an up-hill struggle within such a deprived climate, and seldom necessitates addressing local needs on a priority basis. Maximising the use of health care professionals in specialist fields can prove to be beneficial in terms of conserving the already limited resources while promoting quality of care.

An effective practitioner is an individual who is very knowledgeable about the organisational structure in which he/she works. Only with such knowledge can the practitioner manage effectively and negotiate successfully for the organisation. Cross-cultural health care provision needs to be preceded by systematic cultural assessments to avoid the risks of racial stereotyping while taking into account the values of the community it is intended to serve (Simmons *et al.* 1991). The complex need of clients cared for brings the DM in contact with a variety of health care professionals with whom a network develops – a necessity for negotiating for health care delivery systems.

The DM works as part of a multi-disciplinary team. While the responsibility of each team member is varied, it remains closely inter-related. Effective communication within the team is required to ensure safety and continuity of care. Continually high standards of care can be achieved if a team is effective, bearing in mind that ineffectiveness will result adversely (Quick 1992).

Ongoing Management

Although one of the main focal points of the role of the DM is co-ordinating the effective management of the diabetic clinic, she is also responsible for many other issues relating to the management of all pregnant mothers with abnormal blood glucose levels and the continuing development of the service.

In addition to the GDM clients detected through OGTT are clients with impaired glucose tolerance (IGT). Although a policy is in place to manage clients who fall into the latter group, the provision currently in place remains insufficient and inadequate to cope with the influx of these clients, especially those who fall into the lower scale of *abnormality.* Extra resources need to be invested in the management of this group, as research evidence suggest that these clients, if not managed appropriately, may go on to develop GDM (Pickup and Williams 1991). The recent change in policy which states that random glucose testing should be offered to all pregnant mothers as well as a 16 and 28 weeks OGTT to high risk women places a great strain on the already limited phlebotomy service. Having resources channelled into this area will be useful.

The role of the DM is new and developing. Consequently, the DM is in a key position at this embryonic stage to negotiate successfully for further development of the service. Part of such development includes negotiating for the establishment of a pre- conceptual care clinic for known diabetics and a subsequent evidence based policy to support this clinic.

Domain VI – Monitoring and Ensuring the Quality of Health Care Practice

Immediate Management

When compared to other disciplines, obstetrics is a high-risk speciality that accounts for the highest proportions of legal claims (James 1991). A proactive approach to care management will not only provide higher standards of care, but also reduce the likelihood of adverse outcomes by controlling risks. For this to be successful, it is essential that the care provided by the DM reflects an understanding of GDM and its associated risks while fostering knowledge and experience to effectively co-ordinate the management of those risks relevant to the local population, whether directly or indirectly. Expert help depends on a meaningful engagement in that given situation (Benner 1984). This can be manifest through appropriate referral, staff education through formal and informal teaching, acting as a resource centre for feed-back and support and being available as a medium for effective communication between the obstetric and medical team.

As is customary, a risk card was made, containing biographical details and a social and medical/obstetric history inclusive of Mrs G.'s diagnosis. The card was updated as needed with all complications and admissions. Time was also spent collating data around the labour and delivery to assess the outcome of care. Clients are usually debriefed about the care they received antenatally through to the postnatal period. Even a rudimentary level of client involvement in the evaluation process stimulates a prospect for change (Phillips *et al.*

1994). That information is later used to update the GDM database that is currently formulated for research purposes, with the view to promoting quality standards of care, especially to the local population.

All clients with abnormal blood glucose levels have, added to their pregnancy book pink identifiable stickers to alert staff about the special needs of clients, in order to aid continuity of care and to maintain quality of service. Additionally, special pink sheets are inserted for recording all information relevant to the management of their condition. In fulfilling her professional role of record keeping (Dimond 1994), the DM ensures the use of these sheets by all relevant professionals. Quality of care can only be measured if it can be observed, and omissions in the records may indicate a deficit of care in any stage of the nursing/midwifery process (Newton 1991). In addition to promoting continuity of care, the uniform colour-coded sheets alert professionals to the status of clients with which they are dealing, thus providing timely and appropriate management. This may include referral of clients to other professionals for specialist advice and treatment.

The impact derived from having a *midwife* as part of the obstetric/medical diabetic team, cannot go unnoticed. Success can be measured by the early referral of clients to the diabetic clinic and early attention being paid to diabetic-related issues during pregnancy, and childbirth. The number of clients detected with abnormal blood glucose levels through the increase in appropriate screening and the uptake of postpartum OGTT are significant. The increased interest shown by many to learn about GDM, and its management and the development of the local service provided, continue to act as fuel for growth and development.

Ongoing Management

Midwifery in the future will have new hallmarks (DoH 2000) and changes will be required in its organisation and context of care in order that the recommendations made in the NHS Plan (DoH 2000) can be implemented. With this objective in mind, members of the diabetic team can employ strategic planning to work towards the same goals when caring for women with GDM.

There is a growing interest in the notion of *clinical benchmarking* (DoH 2001), as each Trust strives to market itself as *a* place of excellence, in order to attract purchasers of health care. The provision of evidence based care for women with GDM will be one way for a Trust to demonstrate its commitment to its statutory duty by making the provision of an excellent service to these women one of its top priorities. Women's services and diabetes care are areas highlighted by the local Trust as key targets for improvement for the year 2001. One may, therefore, logically conclude that gestational diabetic care and management will continue to receive great focus.

A dearth of literature supports the need for quality research and auditing to monitor and ensure the quality of health care practice (Dunning *et al.* 1998;

Garcia *et al.* 1998; Lees 1996; Phillips *et al.* 1994; Wright 1989). Bearing in mind the similar effects and management of women with GDM to that of overt diabetics, further research in this area will be invaluable. These research findings can only be beneficial in providing optimal care for a wider cross-section of women who fall into high risk categories.

Auditing the outcome of care for local GDM clients has recently commenced in Newham. At the moment it is difficult to ascertain the true outcome of care. However, based on pure observation, it seems logical to conclude positively in favour of those outcomes. Research into midwifery practice, and validation of it, can be conducted successfully in cases where practices and assumptions are well articulated and can subsequently be tested (Benner 1984). Benner postulates that nurses/midwives do not value their observational powers and clinical experience sufficiently to participate in systematic programmes of data collection, from which credible pieces of research can be derived to inform and develop future practice.

Conclusion

Gestational diabetes mellitus is a major and growing health problem in Newham. Plans for the prevention, identification and effective management of GDM, and particularly its complications, should be formulated at local, national and international levels. It is within the power of bodies at these levels, with specialist help and support, to create conditions in which quality evidence based care can be continuously delivered.

The Borough of Newham has rich cultural diversity. Hence individualised care is paramount. For example, one might have assumed that Mrs G., having immigrated to Britain only two years ago would not have had a good command of the English language and that this would impact on her care. Attention to the details of managing GDM is crucial. For Mrs G., care was appropriate and timely, yielding a positive outcome for her and her baby. The complications associated with GDM were avoided. Mrs G. had a safe, non-traumatic vaginal delivery. Her baby was not macrosomic and, therefore, did not require active therapy. Mrs G. expressed great satisfaction in the care she received. It can be postulated that the standard of care received was exemplary and that this can be used as an acceptable benchmark when caring for others.

The way a woman is cared for relates not only to the history of midwifery and obstetrics. There are many aspects that form a complex framework by which a woman's care can be analysed. A woman does not give birth in a void – laws, professional codes, religious sanctions, cultural traditions and political affiliations all influence women's choices in childbirth. These factors may impact positively or negatively on midwifery care provision and delivery, and will determine the similarities and differences in practice between individuals. Thus, an understanding of the health beliefs, customs and values of each client is an important prerequisite for appropriate care planning and delivery. In order to be effective, and provide optimal care, midwives may at times be obliged to put aside their own notions of what is appropriate for a desired outcome so that clients may feel secure in the knowledge that differences are respected.

References

Abraha, A., C. Schultz, T. Konopelska-Bahu, T. James, A. Watts, I. Stratton, D. Matthews and D. Dunger (1999) 'Glycaemic control and familial factors determine hyperlipidaemia in early childhood diabetes', *Diabetic Medicine*, 16(3) pp. 598–604

Aggleton, P. and H. Chalmers (1989) 'Nursing Models: next year's models', *Nursing Times*, 85(51) pp. 20–7

Akter, J., R. Qureshi, F. Rahim, S. Moosvi, A. Rehman, A. Jabbar, N. Islam and M. Khan (1996) 'Diabetes in Pregnancy in Pakistani Women: Prevalence and Complications in an Indigenous South Asian Community', *Diabetic Medicine*, 13(2) pp. 189–91

Ales, K. and D. Sanitini (1989) 'Should all pregnant women be screened for gestational glucose intolerance?', *Lancet*, 1(8648) pp. 1187–91

Aslam, M., S. Davis and M. Healy (1979) 'Heavy metals in some Asian medicines and cosmetics', *Public Health*, 93(5) pp. 274–84

Aslam, M. and I. Stockley (1979) 'Interaction between curry ingredient (karela) and drug (chlorpropamide)', *The Lancet*, 1 (8116) p. 607

Barker, D. and C. Martyn (1992) 'The maternal and fetal origins of cardiovascular disease', *Epidemiology Community Health*, 46(1) pp. 8–11

Benner, P. (1984) *From Novice to Expert – Excellence and Power in Clinical Nursing Practice*, Menlo-Park, Addison-Wesley Publishing Company

Buchanan, M. (1995) 'Enabling patients to make informed decisions', *Nursing Times*, 91(18) pp. 27–9

Bushard, K., I. Buch, L. Molsted-Pederson, P. Hougaard and C. Khul (1987) 'Increased incidence of true Type-1 diabetes acquired during pregnancy', *British Medical Journal*, 294(6567) pp. 275–9

Chopra, R., I. Chopra, K. Handa and L. Kaper (1958) 'Chopra's Indigenous Drugs of India, Calcutta', Cited, in M. Aslam and I. Stockley (1979), 'Interaction Between curry ingredient (karela) and drug (chlorpropmide)', *The Lancet*, 1(8116) p. 607

De A., J. Soares, A. Dornhorst and R. Beard (1997) 'The case for screening for gestational diabetes', *British Medical Journal*, 315(7110) pp. 737–9

Department of Health (2000) *The NHS Plan: a plan for investment, a plan for reform*, London, The Stationery Office (CM 4818–I)

Department of Health (2001) *The Essence of Care: Patient- focused benchmarking for health care practitioners*, London, The Stationery Office

Dimond, B. (1994) *The Legal Aspects of Midwifery*, London, Haigh and Hochland Publications Limited

Dornhorst, A., P. Bailey, V. Anyaoku, R. Elkeles, D. Johnston and R. Beard (1990) 'Abnormalities of glucose tolerance following gestational diabetes', *Quarterly Journal of Medicine*, 284(77) pp. 1219–28

Dornhorst, A., C. Patterson, J. Nicholls, J. Wadsworth, D. Chiu, R. Elkeles, D. Johnston and R. Beard (1992) 'High prevalence of gestational diabetes in women from ethnic minority groups', *Diabetic Medicine*, 9(9) pp. 820–5

Dornhorst, A. and M. Rossi (1998) 'Risk and prevention of Type-2 diabetes in women with gestational diabetes', *Diabetes Care* (August) 21, Supplement 2, pp. 43–9

Dunning, M., G. Abi-Aad, D. Gilbert, S. Gillam and H. Livett (1998) *Turning Evidence into Everyday Practice*, London, King's Fund Publishing

Enkin, M., J. Marc, K. Renfrew and J. Neilson (1995) *A Guide to Effective Care in Pregnancy and Childbirth*, Oxford, Oxford University Press

Fraser, R. and C. Bruce (1999) 'Amniotic fluid insulin levels identify the foetus at risk of neonatal hypoglycaemia', *Diabetic Medicine*, 16(7) pp. 568–72

Garcia, J., M. Redshaw, B. Fitzsimons and J. Keene (1998) *First Class Delivery – A national survey of women's views of maternity care*, United Kingdom Audit Commission

Hawthorne, K. (1990) 'Asian diabetics attending a British hospital clinic: a pilot study to evaluate their care', *British Journal of General Practice*, 40(6) pp. 243–7

Hawthorne, K., M. Mello and S. Tomlinson (1993) 'Cultural and Religious Influences in Diabetes Care in Great Britain', *Diabetic Medicine*, 10(1) pp. 8–12

Hawthorne, K. and S. Tomlinson (1999) 'Pakistani Moslems with Type-2 diabetes mellitus: effect of sex, literacy skills, known diabetic complications and place of care on diabetic knowledge, reported self-monitoring management and glycaemic control', *Diabetic Medicine*, 16(7) pp. 591–7

Henley, A. (1979) *Asian Patients in Hospital and at Home*, London, King's Fund Publishing Office

Henry, O., N. Beischer, M. Sheedy and J. Walstab (1993) 'Gestational diabetes and follow-up among immigrant Vietnam- born women, Australia and New Zealand', *Journal of Obstetetrics and Gynaecology*, 33(1) pp. 109–14

Hounsome, B. (1998) 'Home blood glucose monitoring', *Professional Nurse*, 13(11) pp. 765–6, 768, 770

James, C. (1991) *Risk management in obstetrics and gynecology*, London, The Medical Defense Union, pp. 36–8

James, D., M. Chiswick, A. Harkes, M. Williams and V. Tindall (1984) 'Maternal diabetes and neonatal respiratory distress: maturation of fetal surfactant', *British Journal of Obstetetrics and Gynaecology*, 91(4) pp. 316–24

Jarrett, R. (1993) 'Gestational diabetes: a non-entity?' *British Medical Journal*, 306(6869) pp. 37–8

Jarrett, R. (1997) 'Should we screen for gestational diabetes?' *British Medical Journal*, 315(7110) pp. 736–9

Jornsay, D., M. Smith-Levintin and B. Petrikovsky (1997) 'Diabetes in pregnancy: How to manage? Part 1: screening and counselling. Part II: antepartum management. Part IV: Labour and delivery', London, *National Intensive Care Publication*, 10(4) pp. 45–50

Khandelwal, M., C. Homko and E. Reece (1999) 'Gestational diabetes mellitus: controversies and current opinions', *Current Opinion in Obstetrics and Gynaecology*, 11(2) pp. 157–65

Kjos, S., R. Peters, A. Xiang, O. Henry, M. Montoro and T. Buchanon (1995) 'Predicting future diabetes in Latino women with gestational diabetes', *Diabetes*, 44(5) pp. 586–91

Kubler-Ross, E. (1984) *On Death and Dying*, London, Tavistock Publications

Kyne-Grzebalski, D., M. Caraher and S. Marshall (1994) 'Diabetes and Pregnancy', *Diabetic Nursing*, 4(1) pp. 2–5

Lavender, T. S. Walkinshaw and I. Walton (1999) 'A prospective study of women's views of factors contributing to a positive birth experience', *Midwifery*, 15(1) pp. 40–6

Lees, P. (1996) *Navigating the NHS – core issues for clinicians*, Oxford, Radcliff Medical Press

Manson, J., E. Rimm, M. Stampher, G. Colditz, W. Willett and A. Krolewski (1991) 'Physical activity and incidence of NIDDM women', *Lancet*, 338(8770) pp. 774–8

Maresh, M., R. Beard, C. Bray, R. Elkeles and J. Wadsworth (1989) 'Factors predisposing to and outcome of gestational diabetes: Part 1', *Obstetrics and Gynaecology*, 74(3) pp. 342–6

Matthews, A. (1993) *In Charge of the Ward*, Oxford, 3rd edn, Blackwell Scientific Publications

McAllister, G. and M. Farquhar (1992) 'Health Beliefs: a cultural division?' *Journal of Advanced Nursing*, 17(12) pp. 1447–54

Metzger, B., N. Cho, S. Roston and R. Radvany (1993) 'Pre-pregnancy weight and antepartum insulin secretion predict glucose tolerance five years after gestational diabetes mellitus', *Diabetes Care*, 16(12) pp. 1598–1605

Monaghan, A., J. Hurst and C. Cox (2000) *Leading Empowered Organisations*, Minnesota, Creative Healthcare Management

Nelson-Piercy, C. and E. Gale (1993) 'Do we know how to screen for gestational diabetes? Current practice in one regional health authority', *Diabetic Medicine*, 11(5) pp. 493–8

Newton, C. (1991) *The Roper-Logan-Tierney Model in Action*, Basingstoke, Macmillan Education Ltd

Niven, A. (1992) *Psychological Care for Families: Before and After Birth*, London, Butterworth Heinemann Ltd

O'Sullivan, J., C. Mahan, D. Charles and R. Dandrow (1973a) 'Gestational diabetes and perinatal mortality rate', *American Journal of Obstetetrics and Gynecolology*, 116(7) pp. 901–4

O'Sullivan, J., C. Mahan, D. Charles and R. Dandrow (1973b) 'Screening criteria for high risk gestational diabetic parents', *American Journal of Obstetetrics and Gynecolology*, 116(7) pp. 895–900

O'Sullivan, J. (1982) 'Body weight and subsequent diabetes mellitus', *JAMA*, 248(8) pp. 949–52

O'Sullivan, J. (1984) 'Subsequent morbidity among gestational diabetic women', in H. Sutherland and J. Stowers (eds), *Carbohydrate metabolism in pregnancy and the newborn*, Edinburgh, Churchill Livingstone, pp. 174–80

Parfitt, V., J. Clark, G. Turner and M. Hartog (1993) 'Use of Fructosamine and Glycated Haemoglobin to verify self blood glucose monitoring data in diabetic pregnancy', *Diabetic Medicine*, 10(2) pp. 162–6

Pettitt, D., K. Aleck, H. Baird, M. Carraher, B. Bennet and W. Knowler (1988) 'Congenital susceptibility to NIDDM: role of the intrauterine environment', *Diabetes*, 37(5) pp. 622–8

Phillips, C., C. Palfrey and P. Thomas (1994) *Evaluating Health and Social Care*, Basingstoke, Macmillan Press Ltd

Pickup, J. and G. Williams (1991) *Textbook of Diabetes* Vol. 2, Oxford, Blackwell Scientific Publication

Quick, T. (1992) *Success Team Building*, London, Amacom

Raphael-Leff, J. (1991) *Psychological Process of Childbearing*, London, Chapman Hall.

Robinson, R. and A. Thompson (1991) *Midwives Research And Childbirth*, Vol. 1, London, Chapman Hall

Rosenstock, I. (1972) 'The health belief model and preventative health behaviour, Health Education Monographs', Vol. 2, cited in K. Hawthorne and S. Tomlinson (1999) 'Pakistani Moslems with Type-2 diabetes mellitus: effect of sex, literacy skills, known diabetic complications and place of care on diabetic knowledge, reported self-monitoring management and glycaemic control', *Diabetic Medicine*, 16(5) pp. 591–7

Saunders, R. and A. James (1985) *The principles and practice of ultrasonography in obstetrics and gynecology*, 3rd edn, Norwalk, Appleton-Century-Crofts,

Sen, D. (1989) 'Asian Culture and Communications in Midwifery', *Midwife, Health Visitor and Community Nurse*, 25 (1 and 2) Jan/Feb pp. 16,18

Silverman, B., B. Metzger, N. Cho and C. Leob (1995) 'Impaired Glucose Tolerance in adolescent offspring of diabetic mothers – Relationship to fetal hyperinsulinism', *Diabetes Care*, 18(5) pp. 611–17

Simmons, D., D. Williams and M. Powell (1989) 'Prevalence of diabetes in predominantly Asian community: preliminary findings of the Coventry diabetes study', *British Medical Journal*, 298(6665) pp. 18–21

Simmons, D., K. Meadows and D. Williams (1991) 'Knowledge of Diabetes in Asians and Europeans With and Without Diabetes: The Coventry Diabetes Study', *Diabetic Medicine*, 8(7) pp. 651–6

Singh-Bhopal, R. (1986) 'The inter-relationship of Folk, Traditional and Western Medicine within an Asian Community in Britain', *Social Science Medicine*, 22(1) pp. 99–105

Sulimani, R., F. Famuyiwa and M. Laajam (1988) 'Diabetes Mellitus and Ramadan Fasting: the need for a critical appraisal', *Diabetic Medicine*, 5(6) pp. 589–91

Trevelyan, J. (1994) 'A Woman's Lot', *Nursing Times*, 90(15) pp. 48–50

UKCC (1993) *Professional Code of Conduct*, London, United Kingdom Central Council for Nursing, Midwifery and Health Visiting

UKCC (1998) *Midwives Rules and Code of Practice*, London, United Kingdom Central Council for Nursing, Midwifery and Health Visiting

Watkins, P. (1998) 'Pregnancy in diabetes: success or failure?' *Diabetic Medicine*, 15(2) p. 95

Watson, J. (1999) *Postmodern Nursing and Beyond*, Edinburgh, Churchill Livingstone

Weeks, J., C. Major, M. deVeciana and M. Morgan (1994) 'Gestational diabetes: does the presence of risk factors influence perinatal outcome?' *American Journal of Obstetetrics and Gynecology*, 171(4) pp. 1003–7

Wright, S. (1989) *Changing Nursing Practice*, London, Edward Arnold

CHAPTER 8

Alteration in Comfort: Caring for the Patient Using Complementary Therapies

CAROL LYNN COX

Patient Profile

Miss M. is a 45 year-old Chinese female, who visited her consultant to obtain a referral for complementary therapies. Miss M. has metastatic carcinoma of the cervix, which has been treated with chemotherapy and radiation therapy. The cancer has now spread to her entire axial skeleton and traditional, Western orthodox medicine has no other treatments that will be effective in the management of her condition. Miss M. is well educated and has a relatively high income. She has been reading recently about the use of complementary therapies, particularly in relation to palliative care and thinks that complementary therapies may assist her in feeling more comfortable. Her consultant is aware that the use of complementary therapies is a growing trend in Great Britain and that a major advantage of complementary therapies is their lack of side effects. Although there have been relatively few studies on the use of complementary therapies in the treatment of cancer, the consultant knows that according to the best data available, complementary therapies are being used extensively in the care of cancer patients in hospices. The consultant referred Miss M. to a Clinical Nurse Specialist (CNS) who specialises in the administration of complementary therapies in palliative care.

Risk Factors

Complementary therapies appear attractive to patients because of the perception that complementary therapies are natural and non-toxic. However some therapies are extremely toxic and may cause multiple complications. It is not always in the best interests of the patient for the doctor to recommend complementary therapies for some types of health problems. In relation to cancer, some complementary therapies have been demonstrated to be of benefit to patients. Therapies used are those that are not harmful by being toxic or cause multiple complications. Indeed, some complementary therapies have been shown to be a source of comfort to the patient. Many patients with cancer or other life-threatening health problems will decide to try complementary therapies. It is critical therefore, that the doctor and CNS discuss honestly and openly with patients their feelings about using complementary therapies and to make every effort possible to ensure that patients are knowledgeable about the types of therapies that will improve their quality of life while being unlikely to produce any harm.

Chief Complaint

Miss M. told the CNS that conventional therapy was no longer helping her feel comfortable. Miss M. was unable to sleep because she felt anxious and was experiencing chronic pain that was no longer being controlled by the medications prescribed by her consultant. She knew that she would be receiving more chemotherapy and radiotherapy and felt that complementary therapies would help her feel less anxious and more comfortable while the chemotherapy and radiotherapy were being administered. Miss M. indicated that she wanted to feel in control of her care and wanted input into the decision making associated with the therapies she would receive. She said she felt a loss of control when decisions were being made about her conventional treatment for cancer.

Background to Recommending Complementary Therapies

The role of the CNS and Nurse Practitioner (NP) in relation to the use of complementary therapies in their practice is an important area for these specialists to consider. The National Health Service's (NHS) present initiatives are targeted towards economic rationalisation and efficiency while providing clinically effective care to patients. The NHS has indicated that in order to meet the needs of patients, health care initiatives must be high quality, cost effective and based on the best evidence available. Government white papers such as the *New NHS Modern and Dependable Services* (Department of Health 1997) and *A First Class Service: Quality in the New NHS* (Department of Health 1998) clarify the NHS's position in relation to the provision of care. Research has indicated that there is a growing population of patients using complementary therapies (BMA 1993). Patients are shifting towards the use of complementary therapies as a way of promoting their own health (Bryne 1995; Mackereth, 1998). Therefore, it is important for the CNS and NP to consider how therapies that are being used by patients or being requested for use by patients can be integrated into their practice. Complementary therapies have been shown to be a cost effective way of providing adjuncts to traditional medical approaches to care. In this chapter information is provided on a variety of complementary therapies used by patients today who are being treated for cancer. The information is underpinned with appropriate evidence upon which the CNS and NP can base their practice. As specialist practice continues to evolve, it is essential that the CNS and NP reflect critically on the health care trends that are shaping society. In order to place this in context, some historical information is provided on each therapy as well as recent developments that have been explicated in the literature. Recent progress in therapeutics and the growing integration of complementary or natural, gentle therapies – as they are known – into healthcare are considered in relation to the cancer patient. There is a focus on the reduction of anxiety and the promotion of comfort, rather than cure.

Western medicine, according to Sasaki (1992) provides many remedies for the problems and diseases people encounter in their lives, however Western medicine concentrates primarily on illness and fails to address the essence of health. Therefore, it may be postulated that modern medicine falls short of many peoples needs when complementary therapies are not integrated with traditional approaches to medicine. Many complementary therapies are identified as systems of medicine, for example, acupuncture, homeopathy and herbalism. This is in contrast to treatments such as iridology, which is considered a diagnostic tool, whereas massage and aromatherapy are considered therapeutic interventions (Rankin-Box 1991). Complementary therapies can be defined as therapies which build upon the therapeutic relationship and address the physical, emotional, mental, psychological and spiritual dimensions of a person's condition (McMahon and Pearson 1991).

The BMA suggested in 1993 that approximately 180 different types of complementary therapies are used by the public in the UK (Bryne 1995). An increase in use of complementary therapies throughout the UK has meant that care must embrace not only traditional Western views about healthcare treatments but also complementary therapies which are derived, in the main, from Eastern perspectives about the promotion of health and the development of a sense of well being. In 1993, Cameron-Blackie identified that the MORI poll of 1989 showed three out of four people surveyed thought complementary therapies should be available through the NHS and further, that a survey conducted by the National Association of Health Authorities and Trusts (NAHAT) in 1992, indicated that the majority of purchasers of health care were in favour of some or all complementary therapies being available on the NHS (Cameron-Blackie 1993). There is a growing awareness among the public of the limitations of orthodox medical care and the side effects of treatment (Leddy and Pepper, 1993) that has led to the recent trend of people integrating complementary therapies with conventional/traditional medicine. It is postulated this leads to a holistic approach to care.

Over the past decade healthcare providers, in particular GPs, have recognised that complementary therapies are beneficial and are presently integrating the use of complementary therapies into their practice. GPs are integrating acupuncture, homeopathy, massage and other therapies into their practices in order to provide a more holistic approach to their patients' care. In conjunction with this, programmes of health education and promotion, which include the use of complementary therapies are being adopted by practice nurses, health visitors and district nurses who are linked to practices through Primary Care Trusts. The aim to promote holistic health has led to the integration and provision of complementary therapies within the NHS. Nurses in the hospital setting are using aromatherapy to promote rest (Price 1998; Price and Price 1995; Stevensen 1994, 1995) and various forms of massage to reduce anxiety, promote sleep and provide comfort (Cox and Hayes 1997, 1998; Richards, 1998).

It has been recognised that many conditions cannot be cured, like that of Miss M., through orthodox medicine. This recognition is fuelling an interest to integrate complementary therapies into the provision of care as these are viewed as gentle, safe and more natural way of reducing anxiety and promoting comfort when cure cannot be achieved. Complementary therapies are considered to have less risk of causing harm to people who use them. Unlike traditional approaches in which synthetic, refined medicines are prescribed by doctors, the treatments employed by complementary therapists are generally derived from natural sources. Many doctors who embrace holistic perspectives find the integration of natural products into their treatment modalities compelling.

A number of medical products that are traditionally given to patients, for example lanoxin, have toxic side effects. Complementary therapies, by and large, involve treatments that are externally applied to the patient, and in instances where substances are taken internally, these substances are natural products that have been diluted to such a finite degree that they are regarded as non-toxic.

There are many types of complementary therapies that could be included in this chapter. However, some of these therapies such as iridology, macrobiotics, naturopathy and spiritual healing have not demonstrated clinical effectiveness through research. Only those therapies that have been demonstrated to be clinically effective for use with cancer patients are addressed.

Definition of the Problem – Pathophysiology

Cervical cancer frequently occurs in women with multiple sex partners, women who began sexual activity before the age of 18 and women whose partners have multiple female partners (Taylor *et al.* 1989). The woman with cervical cancer may be asymptomatic or may experience vaginal bleeding or spotting. Its diagnosis is by Pap smear, and treatment involves surgical removal of the cervix and other surrounding structures if severe. In some instances cryosurgery and laser treatment is used. Pain syndromes in patients with cancer may develop due to the progression of the disease, as a result of the treatment directed at the cure or control of the disease. Pain associated with cancer may be acute or chronic in nature. Acute pain is rapid in onset and varies in intensity from mild to servere. It may last from a very brief intensity up to any period less than six months. When pain lasts longer than six months it is considered chronic. Chronic pain may be intermittent or persistent.

Pain associated with cancer is termed chronic malignant pain (Taylor *et al.* 1989). Bonica (1980) noted that pain associated with cancer has a greater physiologic and psychological impact on a patient than non-cancer chronic pain. Persons with cancer have a greater physical deterioration which is associated with loss of appetite, nausea vomiting and sleep disturbances. In addition, Bonica (1980) indicates that patients with cancer develop greater emotional reactions of anxiety, depression, hypopochondriasis, somatic focusing and neuroticism than patients suffering from chronic pain who do not have cancer. Furthermore, the effects of uncontrolled cancer pain can lead to interpersonal problems, family stress, loss of employment and feelings of dependency and uselessness (Bonica 1980).

Domain I – Management of Client Health/Illness Status

In Domain I the CNS/NP is seen as a direct provider of care. The CNS/NP synthesises theoretical, scientific and contemporary clinical knowledge for the assessment and management of the health and illness of the patient. The domain incorporates illness management in an interdisciplinary context. In the immediate and ongoing management of Miss M.'s health/illness status the CNS played an integral role in co-ordinating the care Miss M. received. In the immediate management phase, care included acupuncture and Chinese herbal medicine.

Immediate Management

Acupuncture

Acupuncture has been identified as an effective treatment for cancer patients experiencing chronic malignant pain. The word acupuncture is derived from the Latin acus (needle) and punctura (puncture). Acupuncture is considered to be an ancient Chinese treatment rooted in Confucian and Taoist philosophy refined over 2000 years ago. Daoist and Taoist philosophy deal with lifestyle and behaviour. These philosophies are designed to encourage moderation, harmony and balance in all things. The actual origin of acupuncture is not known, although excavations in China have revealed stone needles dating back to 3000BC. In the second century BC it was the dominant therapeutic technique employed in China (Unschuld 1985) working from the outside of the body inward. As time passed, the primary theories associated with acupuncture became related to concepts of energy flowing in meridian systems. Acupuncture forms a large part of traditional Chinese medicine. Within the last three decades there has been an increased acceptance and incorporation of acupuncture within traditional Western medicine. The BMA recognizes acupuncture as a discrete clinical discipline (BMA 1993).

Acupuncture involves the insertion of fine sterile needles into specific points on the body. According to Downey (1995), central to the theory associated with acupuncture is the concept of the human body as self-healing and self-rectifying. The body is a dynamic whole; a network of interrelating and interacting energies which through even distribution and flow maintains health (Firebrace and Hill 1988). Conventionally trained healthcare providers postulate acupuncture works within the nervous system by releasing endorphins. Endorphins are hormones which are naturally produced opiates. These practitioners also postulate acupuncture is associated with the *gate theory*, described by Melzak and Wall in 1965, in which physiological gates along the spinal cord open or close in relation to transmission of pain along nerve fibres. Acupuncture acts by stimulating other nerve fibres thus blocking the transmission of pain signals to the brain. As a complementary therapy, it has been shown to be effective in the treatment of pain associated with cancer including post-operative pain management, control of vomiting following chemotherapy and emotional distress. It is administered in a number of different healthcare settings including GP surgeries, in hospital acute care wards, outpatient clinics, hospices, occupational health centres, sports medicine facilities and obstetric wards (in the control of pain associated with labour). Practitioners who perform acupuncture undergo specialised training and take care to ensure in their practice that the whole person is treated rather than providing acupuncture for symptomatic relief alone (Downey 1995).

Acupuncture was prescribed for Miss M. Its use demonstrated effective results in reducing her pain and control of nausea associated with the administration of chemotherapy.

Acupuncture

Acupuncture is a discrete clinical discipline that facilitates the body's self-healing and self-rectifying potential. It has been shown to be effective in the treatment of a variety of diseases and is prescribed to treat the whole person. As a complementary therapy it has been shown to be particularly effective in the treatment and management of pain.

Chinese herbal medicine/herbal medicine

Herbal treatments have been at the centre of medicine throughout history. Recorded practice associated with the use of herbal medicines date back to at least the first century BC in Greece and Egypt and the first Western recording of 455 plants used for medicinal purposes was made by Theophrastus in the third century BC (Griggs 1981). Chinese herbal medicine has been practised for at least 5000 years. Unlike acupuncture that works from the outside in to the body, herbal treatment is posited to work from inside the body outwards. In 1500 BC the Chinese emperor Yen compiled a text on herbal medicine and in AD 200 this text was condensed into a medical text that listed over 350 herbs. This established the basis of Chinese pharmacology. In the sixteenth century the general catalogue of herbs entitled *Li Shi Zheng's Beng Cao Ganu Mu* was written. Chinese herbal medicine is well established and represents one of the fastest growing complementary therapies in the UK.

Chinese herbal medicine and herbal medicine in general employ the properties of a variety of herbs to promote health and prevent illness as well as treat disease. Herbal treatments are prescribed for physical, mental and emotional problems and may be used alone or in conjunction with other complementary therapies. Herbal medicine is considered to be a gentle form of treatment and is postulated to restore balance and harmony to the physical, mental and emotional forces in a person's body. In terms of Chinese medicine, most of the herbs used are exported from China and Taiwan and are dispensed in the UK from Chinese pharmacies.

The World Health Organisation has acknowledged the importance of herbal medicine in terms of treating health problems (WHO 1978). The role of the professional herbalist was identified in the 1968 Medicines Act in the UK. This act makes provision for herbal medicines that cannot be sold over the counter to be prescribed by a professional herbalist. In the UK, the National Institute of Medical Herbalists, which was founded in 1864, regulates standards of practice and training in herbal medicine.

Herbal treatments are based on the premiss that the vital force, or life energy which is known as *Chi* or *Ki* in Chinese medicine, must be in balance and unrestricted in the human body. When this vital force is in balance and circulating freely optimal well-being occurs. Any imbalance or disharmony will result in ill health or disease. In terms of Chinese medicine, there are two opposing forces within *Chi* known as the *Yin* and *Yang*. The forces flow along the channels through which blood or *Xue* flows. When there is an imbalance between the *Yin* and *Yang*, or when the energy flow becomes restricted, balance is lost and disease or illness will occur. *Chi* flows through meridians in the body. Any interruption to this energy flow within the meridians can cause problems to develop in organs that correspond with the meridians. The Chinese herbalist attempts to determine where energy blockages or imbalances occur and then attempts to restore the energy balance through the use of specific herbs.

In terms of integrative therapy within traditional medicine, herbal medicine has a variety of applications. It is considered to be a gentle and highly effective system of health care. Therapeutic effectiveness has been found in treating discomfort and anxiety associated with cancer, cardiovascular problems, migraine headaches, inflammation and various skin conditions (Busby 1995).

The gentle actions of herbal treatment have been shown to promote rest, enhance immunity, act as vasodilators, anti-inflammatory and anti-fungal agents as well as expectorants and mild diuretics (Weiss, 1988; Williams and Home, 1995). For Miss M. the use of herbal medicine in the form of herbal teas was found to be a positive adjunct in promoting rest. In addition Miss M. found the use of herbal medicine congruent with her ethnic background.

Chinese herbal medicine/herbal medicine

Chinese herbal medicine/herbal medicine is well established and has a wide variety of applications. It is one of the fastest growing forms of complementary therapy in the United Kingdom and is regarded as a gentle and highly effective method for promoting health.

Ongoing Management

The CNS/NP must consider therapies that will support the patient over time. Ongoing management may include the use of aromatherapy, homeopathy, reflexology and shiatsu. Each therapy has a specific purpose and has been identified as effective in managing the sequel of cancer.

Aromatherapy

Aromatherapy has been demonstrated to be an effective therapy for promoting a sense of well-being, reducing anxiety and inducing relaxation and sleep in patients who have metastatic carcinoma. It has been estimated that over 40 000 years ago Australian Aborigines were using plant extracts to promote health and a sense of well-being as well as inducing relaxation and sleep. Many of the plant extracts used by Aborigines to treat illnesses are still in use today. Blackwell (1991) and Stevensen (1995) indicate the Australian tea tree, *Maleleuca alternifolia*, which has antibacterial and antifungal properties, was used by Aborigines and is used in aromatherapy today. Six-thousand years ago the Egyptian doctor Imhotep used aromatherapy to facilitate breathing and to stimulate the skin in massage. Essential oils derived from plants have been used by the Hebrews, Greeks and Romans. It is also known that Hippocrates recommended a daily bath scented with oils.

Avicenna, an Arab scholar is attributed with undertaking the first distillation of essential oils in the tenth century. However, Williams (1989) indicates archaeological evidence for the use of essential oils in the Indus Valley civilisation occurred 5000 years earlier. Therapeutic use of essential oils is attributed to R.M. Gattefosse, a French chemist in the early twentieth century. Gattefosse used lavender oil after severely burning his hand in a laboratory accident.

He found that his hand healed quickly and did not scar. Gattefosse published the findings of his research in a text entitled *Aromatherapie* in 1931.

Aromatherapy has been identified as having a distinct therapeutic effect in reducing or alleviating symptoms of distress, thus aiding the person to move towards taking responsibility for managing their own health and wellness (Price and Price 1995). As a form of therapy, it is the fastest growing of all complementary therapies and is used by many nurses and midwives to promote rest, sleep, comfort and reduce anxiety in critical care, acute care, labour and delivery suites, and the hospice environment (Cannard 1994; Price 1998; Stevensen 1994). It has been shown to be an effective treatment when used by patients experiencing side effects from chemotherapy and radiotherapy. The use of aromatherapy in room diffusors and massage became an integral part of Miss M.'s ongoing care that was provided by the CNS.

Homeopathy

The name homeopathy is derived from the Greek words *homios* meaning *like* and *pathos* meaning *suffering*. Homeopathic medicine is produced from natural sources such as plants, metals, minerals, poisonous venoms, insect stings and bacteria. For example, the extract from the common annual belladonna (deadly nightshade) plant, which is frequently found growing on waste ground, quarries and wooded hills throughout central and southern Europe, is used to lessen irritability and treat pain. As a drug belladonna has been found in small doses to allay cardiac palpitations and when used as a plaster applied to the epigastric region relieves discomfort. Belladonna has also been found to be a powerful antispasmodic in treating intestinal colic (Fox 1993).

The principles of homeopathy were known during the time of Hippocrates and are considered to have originated in the fifth century BC. Approximately two-hundred years ago, the German doctor and chemist Samuel Hahnemann (1755–1843) established the modern principles of homeopathy. Hahnemann was concerned that surgical procedures were barbaric and that medicines were given without any sound rationale for their use. He criticised the side effects of many medicines and began experimenting with animal, mineral and vegetable products on human volunteers. Hahnemann developed a taxonomy for each of the products he investigated which was published in the *Law of Similars* in 1796 (Haehl 1985). Central to homeopathy is the view that each person is unique and that each person reacts differently to the same disorder. Hahnemann proposed three essential principles that form the basis of homeopathy today. First, if large doses of a product promote symptoms in a healthy person, then much smaller doses could cure people who have similar symptoms of disease. Second, the *minimum dose* principle was theorised. The *minimum dose* principle states that the greater the dilution of a curative product the more effective it becomes. This theory is known as *potentisation*. Third, the principle of *whole person prescribing* was established. Whole person prescribing means taking into consideration the person's personality, mood, temperament, physical and emotional health, and living conditions. Therefore, although two people may have the same disorder, they may be treated with a different homeopathic medicine.

Homeopathy is a holistic approach to promoting health. Treating like with like stimulates the body to heal itself. Hahnemann referred to this healing as the vital force which through the aid of homeopathic medicines assisted the body in recovering from illness and achieving perfect health. Homeopathic medicines are prepared and dispensed in four basic forms depending on the type of prescription. These are powders, granules, tablets and liquids. The original substance is diluted many times in a water and alcohol base. With each dilution, the liquid is shaken vigorously which is a process known as succussion. Homeopaths postulate this gives the final medicine its power to heal. Dilutions of the substance may be in decimal (1/10th) or centesimal (1/100th) forms. The number of stages in dilution determines the potency of the final product.

The principles of homeopathy are similar to the principles of immunisation, whereby the introduction of a small amount of the substance into the body stimulates the immune system so that when the body is confronted with a disease, health can be maintained. The essential tenet of homeopathic treatment is to tailor the specific treatment to the individual person. Many GPs are trained in the use of homeopathy and prescribe it in conjunction with conventional medicines to promote health. For example, more and more often homeopathic medicine is prescribed to aid in the cessation of smoking. The demand for homeopathic treatment is growing and is one of the complementary therapies available through the NHS. Miss M. was given euphorbium, which is considered to be an effective treatment for pain in terminally ill patients. She was also given cantharis for skin tenderness following radiotherapy.

Reflexology

Reflexology as a practice, derives from an understanding of reflex action of the nervous system. Reflexology is a treatment that involves the application of varying degrees of pressure to focal points on the hands and feet in order to facilitate healing from within. Essentially, the purpose of reflexology is to promote health and a sense of well-being. Approximately 5000 years ago in China and India, as well as among American Indians, various forms of pressure to the feet and hands were used in the treatments of pain and illnesses (Goodwin 1988).

At the end of the nineteenth century, Dr William Fitzgerald, an American ear, nose and throat specialist at Boston General Hospital, discovered that pressure applied to specific points on the hand and foot could cause partial anaesthesia in areas of the ear, nose and throat. Using this technique he performed minor surgical procedures without the aid of conventional anaesthetics. In 1913 Dr. Fitzgerald began to map the zones of the hands and feet and in 1917 in collaboration with a colleague, Dr Edwin Bowers, a text describing *Zone Therapy* was published. Fitzgerald postulated there were ten longitudinal zones running through the body that were related to specific organs. These were reflected on the hands and feet. With controlled pressure, Fitzgerald suggested a response could be produced elsewhere in the body. According to Fitzgerald, reflexology stimulates not only a particular organ associated with the pressure point but also the interrelationship between organs and other body systems. Shortly thereafter in 1920, Dr Joseph Riley further developed the technique and published *Zone Therapy Simplified*. In this text specific horizontal zones of the feet are associated with zone pathways. In the 1960s Doreen Bailey visited America and met Dr Riley's research assistant, Eunice Ingham, who had been refining Riley's technique. Bailey introduced the practice to the UK and established the Bailey's School of Reflexology in 1968.

The theory associated with reflexology suggests every part of the body is connected by pathways which terminate in the soles of the feet, palms of the hands and ears, tongue and head (Ashkenazi 1993; Booth 1994). Reflexologists postulate that the feet are the windows of the body and that they can detect problems in the body by palpating small sand-like grains on the soles of the feet. They indicate these grains are crystalline deposits of calcium located at the end of nerves in the feet. The corresponding areas of the soles of the feet in which they feel the minute grains are related to weak or overactive areas in the body. They claim they can bring about healing by using their thumbs and fingers to rebalance the flow of energy in the zones.

Although there is scepticism as to whether energy can be rebalanced by applying pressure to the foot, many people have indicated they benefit from the therapy. Reflexology is postulated to promote relaxation, and is prescribed for people suffering with chronic diseases like arthritis, anxiety related problems and stress related disorders. According to the Association of Reflexologists, reflexology is designed to boost energy levels and enhance emotional and spiritual well being. The use of reflexology was discussed with Miss M. Although reflexology has been shown to be effective in managing anxiety and stress Miss M. chose not to use this therapy.

Shiatsu

Shiatsu is a Japanese word which means *finger pressure*. It developed from early forms of massage, called *Anma* in Japan, which employ rubbing, stroking, squeezing, tapping, pushing and pulling to influence the muscle tissue and circulatory systems of the body. In contrast to many forms of massage, Shiatsu uses few techniques. It involves the use of gentle manipulation and hand pressure to bring health and vitality into a person's life. To the casual observer it may appear little is happening in terms of physical activity, however through the simple uncomplicated rotation of a limb, or the light pressure of the hand or thumb, it is postulated much is happening internally to the body's energy (Lundberg 1992).

The practice of Shiatsu was developed in the early part of the twentieth century by Tamai Tempaka who was a Japanese medical practitioner. Tamai Tempaka incorporated the Western medical knowledge of anatomy and physiology with gentle manipulation, stretches and pressure to form the practice of Shiatsu. Originally Shiatsu was termed by Tamai Tempaka shiatsu ryoho which means finger pressure way of healing. Over time the terminology changed to shiatsu ho which means finger pressure method, and in 1964 Shiatsu was officially recognized in Japan as a formal therapy by the Japanese government. This recognition distinguished it from the older form of traditional massage, *Anma*. Shiatsu was introduced to the UK about 25 years ago and the Shiatsu Society was founded in 1981.

Central to the principles of Shiatsu is the 2000-year-old philosophy of traditional Chinese medicine. The philosophy states *Tao* or energy is manifested from the universe in the forces of *Yin* and *Yang*; the positive and negative aspects of *Chi* or *Ki*, which flows within the body forming a matrix that links the vital organs with all other parts of the body. *Chi* supports the body and all of its functions. In Chinese treatments the emphasis is on restoring harmony to the *Chi* in the body. *Chi* is considered the primary substance of the universe and arises from the interaction of *Yin* and *Yang*.

Shiatsu is commonly used as a treatment for stress related disorders and for treating back and neck problems. Although there is little scientific evidence that quantify its benefits, one Chinese study found it to be effective in the treatment of chronic low back pain and promoting sleep, and a double blind trial published in the *Journal of the Royal Society of Medicine* indicated Shiatsu improved morning sickness in women attending the Royal Maternity Hospital in Belfast (Jones 1998). Shiatsu was discussed with Miss M. as an approach to the promotion of sleep. However as with reflexology, Miss M. chose not to use this therapy.

Shiatsu

Shiatsu employs the use of hand pressure and gentle manipulation to improve health, vitality and stamina. It is prescribed for many conditions and is regarded as being very relaxing. Through the balancing of the body's energy, it is postulated better physiological and psychological functioning occurs.

Domain II – The Nurse–Client Relationship

The CNSs/NPs profound regard for and commitment to human beings forms the foundation for the use of complementary therapies outlined in Domain II. This commitment is unaltered by social, educational, economic, cultural, racial, religious and other attributes of the patients receiving care, including the nature and duration of disease or illness (NONPF 1995). Domain II typifies the personal, egalitarian, collaborative approach which enhances the clinical effectiveness of care. Interpersonal transaction is collaborative as it relates to the therapeutic regimen that enhances patient outcomes. The interpersonal relationship that is established between the patient and the CNS/NP becomes the vehicle through which patients participate in their care. Expert care manifest in the Nurse–Client Relationship provides the opportunity for the patient to incorporate feelings of self-efficacy and empowerment in relation to choices that are made long term in relation to the patient's care. For Miss M. the following therapies formed a substantial adjunct to self-care.

Immediate Management

Massage and touch

The word massage is derived from the Arabic, Greek, Hindi and French words which describe forms of touch, pressing and shampooing (Horrigan 1995). It is a systematic manipulation of the soft tissues of the body. Regardless of the individual touch technique that has been developed by the massage therapist, manipulations will be gliding, kneading, percussing, compressing, shaking or vibrating.

In an ancient Chinese book *The Cong-Fou of the Tao-Tse*, the techniques of modern massage a described. Approximately one hundred years ago a French translation of the text brought Chinese massage to the Western world. Consequently, although there are now many forms of massage, such as the Swedish movements of massage which were systematised by Per Henrik Ling – a Swedish gymnast in the early nineteenth century – the French terminology for massage strokes is used. Strokes that glide are termed *effleurage*; those that knead are termed *petrissage*; those that percus are termed *tapotement*; those that compress are termed *friction*; and those that shake or vibrate are termed *vibration*.

According to Tappan (1988) massage probably began as soon as the cave dwellers rubbed their bruises. Therapeutic massage undoubtedly developed from local folk medicine and although the origin of Chinese medicine is lost in antiquity, it appears massage has always been an essential aspect of healing. Documents in the British Museum indicate massage was performed in China around 3000 BC (Horrigan 1995). It has been found useful and integral to the healing process and is frequently prescribed for its psychological, physiological, mechanical and reflex effects. Hippocrates learned the art of massage and prescribed it for his patients in 400 BC and Asclepiades, who was an eminent Greek doctor, abandoned the use of all other medicines in favour of massage, which he claimed effected cure by restoring the nutritive fluids of the tissues to their natural, free movement. He discovered that sleep could be induced by gentle stroking. During the First and Second World Wars massage was used extensively to promote physical and emotional rehabilitation in battle worn soldiers. Massage therapy has been embraced by the caring professions and in particular among nurses. In the primary and secondary care sector massage is used extensively in areas such as pain clinics, cancer wards, hospices, care of the elderly units and physiotherapy departments.

Massage has been shown to be effective in promoting sleep and recovery in critically ill patients (Richards 1998). The effects of massage and associated therapeutic touch have been shown to reduce anxiety, promote comfort and rest in the intensive care environment (Cox and Hayes 1997, 1998). Through massage, aspects of sleep deprivation can be ameliorated (Bonnet 1994). Miss M. undertook massage therapy with an essential oil (lavender) in order to reduce her anxiety and promote sleep.

Massage

Massage is considered to be a gentle way of promoting health. It has been shown to be effective in promoting comfort, sleep and recovery as well as reducing feelings of anxiety and stress.

Ongoing Management

Art, music, poetry and dance therapy

From the beginning of time, human beings have engaged in self-expression through forms of art, music, writing and dance. The Hippocratic model of 2000 years ago held that 'there is one flow; one common breathing; all things are in sympathy' (Graham 1991), while 20 000 years ago Shaman healers used dance, drawing and story telling as a means to promote health and well being. Shamans were considered to be holistic practitioners who attempted to harmonise the individual and the environment. Drawing, listening to music, writing poetry and dancing are considered to be gentle, non-invasive forms of caring for the self that instil feelings of relaxation and calmness. In instances where tension and anxiety are experienced over long periods of time, this can have a depressing effect on the immune system leading to ill-health and disease (Ryman 1994). Art therapy, music therapy, dance therapy and reading poetry are activities which provide a form of pleasure which reduces feelings of anxiety and are often prescribed when people experience depression. Music, when used in the coronary care setting, has been shown to reduce anxiety and effect a happier emotional state (Bolwerk 1990; Davis-Rollans and Cunningham 1987). The text *Soulskin* states

> Everything is in resonance. Each note of the scale resonates with the atomic number of one of the elements, with a colour of the spectrum, and with the placement of the planets around the sun. Your body has it note. If your are ill, this note can make you well. If in pain, this note diminishes that pain. (Krysl 1996: 47).

People have indicated, following the diagnosis of cancer, that these therapies have helped them change their lifestyle and gain a sense of well being. Miss M. was encouraged to listen to her favourite music on a regular basis in order to effect a happier emotional state.

Domain – III The Teaching Coaching Function

In this domain, teaching coaching skills include the CNSs ability to impart knowledge and associated psychomotor skills to patients, in order for patients to be self caring. Coaching for Miss M. involved individualising therapies through the activities of modelling and tutoring. When the CNS had identified that Miss M. was ready for integrating more personalised activities into her daily regimen, the CNS instructed her in meditation, *Tai Chi* and yoga techniques.

Immediate Management

Meditation

Meditation is considered to be a hard discipline akin to a good programme of physical exercise (Leshan 1995). It has been practised for over 2000 years in Asia and is documented as a part of the monastic life found in Buddhist monasteries. Maharishi Mahesh Yogi developed transcendental meditation in the early 1960s. This form of meditation was enthusiastically embraced by the flower children of the 1960s. They postulated it brought about a sense of peace and feelings of well being. The Friends of the Western Buddhist Order established a slightly different form of meditation in Britain in 1967 and consequently a large number of British people practise meditation for about 20 minutes once or twice each day. Meditation involves sitting quietly and sweeping away all thoughts from the conscious mind. This frees the unconscious mind to do its work. Many GPs prescribe its use, particularly as a means of reducing anxiety and stress. The British Association for the Medical Application of Transcendental Meditation boasts a membership of over 700 GPs and hospital doctors.

Leshan (1995) indicates people meditate to find, recover or come back to something of themselves that they have lost. It is used as a means of achieving spiritual awareness and fulfilment, as well as a means to reduce or alleviate inner turmoil and feelings of stress. Through its use a deep sense of relaxation occurs. Meditation is designed to improve physical, psychological and spiritual well-being by accessing more of an individual's human potential. It is said to bring the person closer to the self and reality. There are many forms of meditation.

- *Transcendental meditation (TM)* is probably the most popular and is frequently prescribed to reduce stress levels. In order to practise TM the person sits quietly and repeats a personally significant word or *mantra* in their head. The critical element of TM is that the *mantra* or word should either be nonsensical, such as *La Di* or one of a positive nature such as *peace.*
- *Buddhist meditation* is associated with specific breathing techniques associated with the abolition of negative feelings. While employing specific breathing techniques, the person focuses on the replacement of positive, constructive thoughts that are designed to alter attitudes about the self. This form of meditation is postulated to bring about a greater sense of self-worth and spiritual contentment.
- *Mantra meditation* is a technique centred on repeating a basic word or sound. The mind drifts without direction. In that a basic word or sound is repeated, mantra meditation is similar to TM. The word or sound should have no meaning whatsoever, and as in Buddhist meditation is intended to free the unconscious mind to do its work. This form of meditation is postulated to produce feelings of tranquillity and serenity.

There are contraindications to meditation. People who are suffering from depression, or have epilepsy or organic psychiatric disorders such as schizophrenia should not meditate unless use of the therapy has been approved by their doctor. Meditation brings about deep states of relaxation. An increase in alpha wave activity, which is normally associated with rest, has been suspect in inducing focal seizures.

Evidence suggests people who meditate indicate they sleep better and experience less anxiety (Leshan 1995). Many people have used meditation as a means to reduce their smoking and drinking habits and it is intriguing to note that many GPs are now using meditation for this purpose. Research associated with TM suggests people who suffer from anxiety, sleeplessness, migraine, tension headache, irritable bowel syndrome, stomach ulcers, asthma and high blood pressure benefit (Jones 1998).

In the text *Journey Into Health, Awakening The Wisdom Within You* a simple meditation is given. It is 'Perfect health, pure and invincible, is a state we have lost. Regain it, and we regain a world.' (Chopra 1995:11). The CNS taught Miss M. a simple mantra to use in meditating. Miss M. was encouraged to meditate for ten minutes daily to reduce her feelings of anxiety and to promote sleep.

Ongoing Management

Tai Chi

In the early morning, before the busy day begins in China, people of all ages begin the day by performing traditional Chinese exercises in parks, woods or where they live. A common sight is *Tai Chi Chuan* which is an exquisite slow exercise, a soft martial art, that develops and relaxes the whole body (Lam 1991). *Tai Chi* originated in the Sung Dynasty of the twelfth century. It was developed by a Taoist monk, Chang San Feng, who was a soldier, spiritualist and martial arts expert. According to legend, Chang San Feng observed a duel between a snake and crane. During the duel the snake mesmerised the crane by its artful speed and grace. Chang San Feng was so impressed by the agility of the snake that he developed a system of non-combative martial art exercises that integrated the snake-like movements with relaxation techniques, breathing exercises and meditation. *Tai Chi* is frequently referred to as a moving meditation.

Tai Chi has grown in popularity since the early 1970s. It is widely practised by men and women in the UK and is regarded as a beautiful and soothing antidote to the stresses and strains of modern life. Although there are many forms of *Tai Chi*, all forms are designed to aid in the flow of vital energy in the body. This helps to establish balance. When practised regularly, *Tai Chi* improves posture, suppleness and respiratory functioning. It stimulates the circulatory and lymphatic systems and promotes relaxation of the nervous and musculo-skeletal systems. Miss M. was encouraged to join a local *Tai Chi* group in her neighbourhood in order to maintain suppleness and respiratory functioning. Miss M. found the therapy so enjoyable she practiced it every morning.

Yoga

In 8000 BC the yoga cult in India used respiratory exercises for religious and healing purposes. The word yoga was derived from the Sanskrit word for *union* that means promoting union between the mind and body. Like *Tai Chi*, yoga is considered as a moving meditation. Although the origins of yoga are unknown, the practice, as known today, probably began about 5000 years ago. It was brought to the UK in the Victorian era and has become increasingly popular since its introduction. Yoga is an exercise system that enhances the *psyche* (mind) and *some* (body). The postures adopted in yoga increase suppleness and strength while inducing relaxation. In practice, yoga alleviates stress and counters negative emotions. Yoga induces an inner calm through concentration on postures (exercises) and breathing. This is postulated to enhance digestion, relieve tension, reduce feelings of anxiety, and bring about spiritual well-being. Yoga is frequently prescribed as a treatment for back pain and depression.

Breathing is central to the philosophy of yoga. Therapeutic effects occur through correct breathing. Anxiety, tension and stress manifest themselves in disorders such as indigestion, irritable bowel syndrome and headaches. Through breathing exercises which use all of the lung and respiratory muscles in expanding the chest, oxygenation of the blood is improved, the involuntary nervous system is stimulated, and energy and vitality are enhanced.

There is considerable evidence that yoga is a valuable form of complementary therapy. In 1985, the *British Medical Journal* indicated regular practice of yoga by asthmatic patients reduced the number of asthmatic attacks they experienced and also reduced the dosage of medication required to manage their symptoms (Jones 1998). Yoga has been used in NHS hospitals and hospices for treatment of the terminally ill as well as treating mylagic encephalomyelitis (ME) and emphysema. Yoga has been shown to be effective in reducing anxiety and other stress related conditions such as palpitations and high blood pressure. Balance and harmony are induced through yoga and this promotes a healthy lifestyle. Miss M. was also encouraged to explore the use of yoga to reduce her feelings of anxiety. However Miss M. enjoyed practicing *Tai Chi* and indicated she had no desire to take up yoga.

Domain IV – Professional Role

In this domain the CNS directed the care Miss M. needed based on a firm foundation of theory and research. From a role perspective, an important competency the CNS maintained was the ability to manage the multiple needs and requests of Miss M. without losing sight of the overall objectives in Miss M.'s care.

Immediate Management

The NHS has indicated that in order to meet the needs of patients, healthcare initiatives must be high quality, cost effective and based on the best evidence available. Complementary therapies can be used in a variety of healthcare contexts to provide high quality clinically effective care to patients. Complementary therapies, when integrated with traditional Western approaches to care, meet the NHS agenda as it relates to an holistic approach to care that is regarded as satisfying to patients. It is recommended that the therapies addressed in this chapter should be considered by the CNS and NP for use in their professional practice. Complementary therapies lead to a less fragmented way of providing care.

The integration of complementary therapies

A growing awareness of the limitations of orthodox medicine and its side effects has led people to integrate complementary therapies into their healthcare regimen. Complementary therapies can be used in conjunction with traditional Western medicine to reduce anxiety and promote comfort in cancer patients experiencing chronic malignant pain. The integration of complementary therapies should be under the direction of a qualified doctor to ensure that there are no contraindications to their use and that the most effective form of therapy is employed.

Domain V – Managing and Negotiating Health Care Delivery Systems and Domain VI – Monitoring and Ensuring the Quality of Health Care Practice

In Domains V and VI the CNS is required to control and/or direct systems of complementary therapies for the patient and to ensure these are delivered safely and are ethically sound. In managing and negotiating health care delivery systems the CNS administers and prescribes complementary therapies to achieve improved healthcare outcomes for the patient. In monitoring and ensuring the quality of healthcare practice, the CNS ensures that standards of conduct associated with the administration of complementary therapies are evidence-based. Clinical governance is foremost in supporting the management of the patient's healthcare.

Clinical governance aims to provide a framework to continuously improve the quality of services in the NHS and safeguard high standards of care by creating an environment in which excellence in clinical care can flourish (DoH 1999a). With the advent of clinical governance, consideration has been given to clinical effectiveness. This is an agenda item that the CNS and NP cannot ignore in relation to their practice. Therefore, as consideration is given to integrating complementary therapies into specialist practice, the specialist must consider the clinically effective nature of the therapy.

As indicated in a publication in the *British Journal of Nursing* (Cox and Ahluwalia 2000) little research in the area of developing clinical effectiveness has been published. There are guidelines and initiatives on developing clinical effectiveness that have been published by the National Health Service Executive (1996) and the Royal College of Nursing (1996). The National Institute for Clinical Excellence (DoH 1999b) provides guidelines for health professionals about the effectiveness of particular interventions for specific patients. The practice of CNS and NP in relation to the use of complementary therapies should be based on the aforementioned guidelines and their interventions built upon the premiss of achieving clinically effective care.

Conclusion

The use of complementary therapies is a growing trend in the UK. In the USA substantial interest in the use of complementary therapies has been identified and therefore, The National Institute of Health in Bethesda, Maryland has developed a centre for the study of potentially beneficial treatments. Some complementary therapies have been identified as being of benefit to patients, even if only in terms of providing the patient, like Miss M., with an intervention that reduces anxiety, promotes comfort and rest, and maintains the patient's sense of hope. The CNS/NP should help the patient discern between harmful therapies and those that are not. The CNS should also ensure that the complementary therapies used serve as an adjunct to traditional Western medicine and do not keep the patient away from proven curative or palliative therapies that may improve quality of life. Miss M. found the use of complementary therapies that were prescribed and administered by her CNS to be of benefit in relation to reducing her anxiety, promoting comfort and enhancing sleep.

References

Ashkenazi, R. (1993) 'Multidimensional reflexology', *International Journal of Alternative and Complementary Medicine*, 6(3) pp. 8–12

Blackwell, A. (1991) 'Tea tree oil and anaerobic (bacterial) vaginosis', *The Lancet*, (Letter) 337(8736) p. 300

BMA (1993) *Complementary medicine*, Oxford, Oxford University Press

Bolwerk, C. (1990) 'Effects of relaxing music on state anxiety in myocardial infarction patients', *Critical Care Nursing Quarterly*, 13(2) pp. 63–72

Bonica, J. (1980) 'Pain research and therapy: Past and current status and future needs', in L. Ng and J. Bonica (eds), *Pain, Discomfort and Humanitarian Care*, Proceedings of the National Conference, NIH, Bethesda, MD, 15–16 February 1979, New York, North Holland, Elsevier

Bonnet, M. (1994) 'Sleep deprivation', in N., Kryger, T. Roth and W. Dement (eds), *Principles and Practice of Sleep Medicine*, 2nd edn, Philadelphia, W.B. Saunders

Booth, B. (1994) 'Reflexology', *Nursing Times*, 90(1) pp. 38–40

Bryne, C. (1995) 'Choosing a therapy', in D. Rankin-Box (ed.), 'The Nurses' Handbook of Complementary Therapies', Edinburgh, Churchill Livingstone

Busby, H. (1995) 'Herbal medicine', in D. Rankin-Box (ed.), *The Nurses' Handbook of Complementary Therapies*, Edinburgh, Churchill Livingstone

Cameron-Blackie, G. (1993) *Complementary Therapies in the NHS*, Brimingham, National Association of Health Authorities and Trusts

Cannard, G. (1994) 'On the scent of a good night's sleep', Trial project, *Midland Health Board News*, January, p. 3

Chopra, D. (1995) *Journey Into Healing Awakening The Wisdom Within You*, London, Rider

Cox, C. and S. Ahluwalia (2000) 'Enhancing clinical effectiveness among clinical nurse specialists', *British Journal of Nursing*, 9(16) pp. 702–10

Cox, C. and J. Hayes (1997) 'Reducing anxiety: the employment of Therapeutic Touch as a nursing intervention', *Complementary Therapies in Nursing and Midwifery*, 3(6) pp. 162–7

Cox, C. and J. Hayes (1998) 'Experiences of administering and receiving Therapeutic Touch in intensive care', *Complementary Therapies in Nursing and Midwifery*, 4(5) pp. 128–33

Davis-Rollans, C. and S. Cunningham (1987) 'Physiologic responses of coronary care patients to selected music', *Heart and Lung*, 16(4) pp. 370–8

Department of Health (1997) *The New NHS Modern and Dependable Services*, London, HMSO

Department of Health (1998) *A First Class Service: Quality in the New NHS*, London, HMSO

Department of Health (1999a) *Clinical Governance: Quality in the New NHS*, Leeds, NHSE

Department of Health (1999b) *National Institute for Clinical Excellence*, London, HMSO

Downey, S. (1995) 'Acupuncture', in D. Rankin-Box (ed.), *The Nurses' Handbook of Complementary Therapies*, Edinburgh, Churchill Livingstone

Firebrace, P. and S. Hill (1988) *New ways to health – a guide to acupuncture*, London, Hamlyn

Fox, A. (1993) 'General practice management of gastrointestinal problems assisted by Vegatest techniques', *British Homeopathic Journal*, 82(1) pp. 87–91

Goodwin, H. (1988) 'Reflex zone therapy', in D. Rankin-Box (ed.), *Complementary health therapies: a guide for nurses and the caring professions*, London, Chapman and Hall

Graham, H. (1991) 'The return of the Shaman: the emergence of a biophysical approach to health and healing', *Complementary Medical Research*, 5(3) pp. 165–71

Griggs, G. (1981) *Green pharmacy: a history of herbal medicine*, London, Jill Norman and Hobhouse

Haehl, R. (1985) *Samuel Hahnemann, His life and work*, Volumes 1 and 2, New Delhi, B. Jain

Horrigan, C. (1995) 'Massage', in D. Rankin-Box (ed.), *The Nurses' Handbook of Complementary Therapies*, Edinburgh, Churchill Livingstone

Jones, H. (1998) *Doctor, What's the Alternative?* London, Hodder and Stoughton

Krysl, M. (1996) 'Sound Healer', in M. Krysl (ed.), *Soulskin*, New York, National League for Nursing

Lam Kam Chuen, Master (1991) *The Way of Energy*, London, Gaia Books Ltd

Leddy, S. and J. Pepper (1993) *Conceptual Bases of Professional Nursing*, 3rd edn, Philadelphia, J. B. Lippincott Company

Leshan, L. (1995) *How to Meditate*, London, Thorsons

Lundberg, P. (1992) *Shiatsu*, London, Gaia Books Ltd

Mackereth, P. (1998) 'Body, relationship and sacred space', *Complementary Therapies in Nursing and Midwifery*, 4(5) pp. 125–7

McMahon, R. and A. Pearson (1991) *Nursing as therapy*, London, Chapman and Hall

National Health Service Executive (1996) *Achieving Effective Practice: A clinical effectiveness and research information pack for nurses, midwives and health visitors*, NHSE, Leeds

NONPF (National Organisation of Nurse Practitioners Faculties Curriculum Guidelines Task Force) (1995) *Advanced Nursing Practice, Curriculum Guidelines and Programme Standards for Nurse Practitioner Education*, Washington DC

Price, S. (1998) 'Using essential oils in professional practice', *Complementary Therapies in Nursing and Midwifery*, 4(5) pp. 144–7

Price, L. and S. Price (1995) *Aromatherapy for health professionals*, Edinburgh, Churchill Livingstone

Rankin-Box, D. (1991) 'Proceed with caution', *Nursing Times*, 87(45) pp. 34–6

Richards, K. (1998) 'Effect of a Back Massage and Relaxation Intervention on Sleep in Critically Ill Patients', *American Journal of Critical Care*, 7(4) pp. 288–99

Royal College of Nursing (1996) *Clinical Effectiveness, A Royal College of Nursing Guide*, Royal College of Nursing, London

Ryman, L. (1994) 'Relaxation and visualisation', in R., Wells and V. Tschudin (eds), *Wells' supportive therapies in health care*, London, Bailliere Tindall

Sasaki, P. (1992) 'Foreword', in P. Lundberg (ed.), *Shiatsu*, London, Gaia Books Ltd

Stevensen, C. (1994) 'The psychophysiological effects of aromatherapy following cardiac surgery', *Complementary Therapies in Medicine*, 2(1) pp. 27–35

Stevensen, C. (1995) 'Aromatherapy', in D. Rankin-Box (ed.), *The Nurses' Handbook of Complementary Therapies*, Edinburgh, Churchill Livingstone

Tappan, F. (1988) *Healing Massage Techniques, Holistic, Classic, and Emerging Methods*, Norwalk, Appleton and Lange

Taylor, C., C. Lillis and P. LeMone (1989) *Fundamentals of Nursing*, London, J.B. Lippincott

Unschuld, P. (1985) *Medicine in China: a history of ideas*, Berkley, University of California Press

Weiss, R. (1988) *Herbal medicine*, Beaconsfield, Beaconsfield Press

Williams, D. (1989) *Lecture notes on essential oils*, London, Eve Taylor

Williams, L. and Home, V. (1995) 'A comparative study of some essential oils for potential use in topical applications for the treatment of the yeast *Candida albicans*', *Australian Journal of Medical Herbalism*, 7(3) pp. 57–62

World Health Organisation (1978) *The promotion and development of traditional medicine*, World Health Organisation technical report series, No. 662, Geneva, WHO

CHAPTER 9

Alteration in Endocrine Function: Caring for the Patient With Leg Ulcers

MICHAEL VAN ORSOUW

Patient Profile

Mr C. was born in St Mary's Hospital, Stratford and has lived in the East End of London all his life. He is a 68 year old Caucasian male who retired as a warehouse worker ten years ago. Single, he never married and lives with sister and brother-in-law in a private house. His hobbies include fishing and football. He currently receives a state pension but no social services assistance.

Risk Factors

Mr C. was diagnosed as being a diabetic in 1952, and had previously been admitted to hospital on three separate occasions with diabetic foot ulcers and for arterial by-pass surgery to both limbs. On each occasion Mr C. self-discharged as he had become frustrated with the length of time the ulcers were taking to heal. In spite of advice to give up smoking, Mr C. continues to smoke 20 cigarettes a day.

Chief Complaint

Mr C. presented with a diabetic foot ulcer and was referred to the vascular nurse specialist by his district nurse who was concerned about the condition of his foot. The district nurse had been dressing the wound for approximately one week; what had started as a small wound on the dorsum of the foot had grown rapidly into a large black necrotic ulcer. Consequently, the Vascular Nurse Specialist arranged a joint visit to the patient's home with the district nurse to make an assessment of the wound, which now showed signs of cellulitis. The Vascular Nurse Specialist arranged an urgent hospital admission via the Accident and Emergency Department at Newham General

Hospital. Mr C. was examined by the vascular team and was admitted to the hospital.

Other Complaints

Having had several previous diabetic foot ulcers Mr C. was well aware that this admission would entail a lengthy stay in hospital. Due to the radical extent of Mr C.'s surgery, he required extensive psychological support to come to terms with the change in his body image and his new footwear. While Mr C. was in hospital his sister became unwell and was admitted to a neighbouring hospital. She unfortunately died, which further affected Mr C.'s psychological demeanour.

Definition of the Problem – Pathophysiology

There are two major factors which are related to the aetiology of foot lesions associated with diabetes. These are neuropathy and peripheral vascular disease which cause lesions that may be complicated by infection.

Neuropathy

Peripheral neuropathy as a complication of diabetes is probably the most common consequence of diabetes. This affects approximately 30 per cent of patients (Kumar *et al.* 1994). Disturbances in metabolism caused by hyperglycaemia (Cotter and Cameron 1997) reduces nerve blood supply, causing damage to the somatic (sensory motor) and autonomic nervous system. Neuropathy is usually progressive and permanent.

An imbalance of the intrinsic muscles causes the foot to become cavus in shape with the metatarsal heads becoming prominent, demonstrating clawing of the toes. The fat pads over the ball of the foot move forward and the foot's natural cushioning is lost. Hyperkeratosis develops as a natural response to pressure. Excess callus which is not debrided regularly can lead to ulceration. Additionally, due to damage to the autonomic nerve system, the feet may not sweat. This results in dry feet that are more likely to crack or fissure and become prone to further callus formation and possible infection.

Patients with sensory loss may loose their protective pain sensation, which may exacerbate any ulceration that may have occurred. Conversely some patients develop a painful neuropathy which can vary from mild paraethesia in a few toes to severe, unremitting pain in both legs (Pavy 1985). If thermal sensation is lost, extremes of temperature may not be felt and the patient may burn their feet without knowing it. Clinically, it is of importance that chemical treatments for corns which can damage healthy skin should not be used.

Peripheral Vascular Disease (PVD)

The vascular component of the disease associated with diabetes occurs in both Type-I and Type-II diabetes but is more common in the former (Renwick *et al.* 1998). The main factor responsible for a reduction in blood supply to the foot is atheosclerosis of the large vessels in the leg. In the diabetic patient it affects the distal vessels, manifesting itself at an earlier stage and tending to be more severe (Laing 1998). Calcification involving the intimal plaque and media is frequent in arteries at all levels in patients with diabetes. This may lead to false pressure readings when monitoring the patients' ankle brachial pressure index (ABPI) (Reiber *et al.* 1998). The earliest symptom of PVD is claudication, or leg pain on walking a given distance. Due to neuropathy the patient may have difficulty describing this pain. Pain at rest or night pain may develop as PVD progresses. If left untreated, tissue ulceration and gangrene will develop (Reiber *et al.* 1998).

It is argued that diabetic patients with an ischaemic foot ulcer commonly have some form of neuropathy, therefore, ulcers in diabetics can be described as neuropathic ulcers (where neuropathy predominates with pulses present) or neuroischaemic ulcer (where there is both neuropathy and an absence of a pulse). The difference between neuropathic ulcers and neuroischaemic ulcers is that neuropathic feet present with warm pink skin and palpable pulses. Whereas neuroischaemic feet present with cool atropic skin and impalpable pulses (Edmonds and Foster 1996). In neuropathic feet the ulcer is painless and digital gangrene may be present. However in neuroischaemic feet the ulcer may be painful and claudication and rest pain are frequent complaints verbalised by the patient. Digital gangrene may also be present (Edmonds and Foster 1996).

Treatment

Treatment options for diabetic foot ulcers depend on the type and location of the ulcer. When diagnosing the ulcer, the difference between neuroischaemic and neuropathic feet should be noted. The assessment of patients with diabetes should begin with a complete history and physical status. Patients may report a history that suggests generalised atheosclerosis, such as a history of coronary heart disease, cerebrovascular accident or claudication. Many patients may have already undergone vascular surgery (Steed 1998). The foot should be evaluated for pulses. If either the dorsalis pedis or posterial tibial pulse can be felt, then the foot is unlikely to have significant ischaemia (Edmonds and Foster 1998). The use of monofilaments which buckle at a force of 10g has been shown to be effective in screening for neuropathy (Kumar *et al.* 1991), with abnormality being associated with a 10-fold increased risk of ulceration, but standardisation and specification have yet to be fully determined (Kumar *et al.* 1996)

Neuropathic Management

The management of neuropathic foot ulcers can be divided into three parts:

1) *Removal of callus*
   Callus is normally removed by a registered chiropodist (podiatrist) using a scalpel to reveal the base of the ulcer. Debridement can also reveal ulceration underneath the callus (Knowles and Jackson 1997).
2) *Eradication of infection*
   Diabetes is well recognized as a risk factor for wound infections (Cruse and Foord 1973). A diabetic foot infection is a *medical emergency.* Early aggressive debriding of necrosis and drainage of the infection is necessary (Rosenblum *et al.* 1994). Any open ulcer on the sole of the foot will be colonised by bacteria; however, only ulcers with deep infection (for example osteomyelitis) or cellulitis require treatment (Laing 1998). Though superficial cellulitis is usually caused by a single pathogen (usually *Staphylococcus auerus* or streptococci), most infections in the diabetic foot are polymicrobic, with three to six organisms typically isolated per infection, as shown below (Caputo 1994).
   - Gram-positive cocci
     - *Staphylococcus aureus*
     - Coagulase-negative staphylococci (S. *epidermidis*)
     - Streptococci
     - Enterococci
   - Gram-negative bacilli
     - Enterobacteriaceae (e.g. *Escherichia colt, Proteus app., Klebsiella, Enterobacter*)
     - *Pseudomonas aeruginosa*
   - anaerobes
     - *Bacteroides spp.*
     - Peptostreptococci

   Antibiotics prescribed to treat diabetic foot ulcers therefore must cover Gram-negative, Gram-positive and anaerobes. To this end, in Newham the following antibiotics are prescribed for severe infections:

   Gentamicin – is given parentally and, although it is relatively inexpensive, the hidden costs in monitoring blood levels and renal function must be considered. Gentamicin has a good spectrum of activity but does not include *Enterococcus spp.*, or anaerobic organisms.

Flucloxacillin – is given parentally with good activity against *Staphylococcus aureus* but gives poor cover for Gram-negative bacilli and anaerobes.

Metronidazole – is usually given rectally and is invaluable in the management of anaerobic foot infections that are commonly found in diabetic ulcers.

Once the infection is less severe, ciprofloxacin is prescribed. This drug is active against a broad spectrum of Gram-positive and Gram-negative organisms, but is inactive against anaerobes, so it is normally given in combination with metronidazole.

3) *Reduction of weight-bearing forces* (Edmonds and Foster 1996)
During an acute stage of ulceration the patient may be nursed on bed rest, to remove weight-bearing forces to promote healing. Care must be taken to protect the neuropathic patient's heels while in bed. When bed rest is not suitable for the patient, they can be managed, in the short term, by using a total contact plaster cast, Scotch cast boot or an air cast boot. For the long-term treatment of neuropathic ulcers, specialised footwear which is fashioned from casts of the patient's foot is required. Prescribed footwear can prevent ulcer recurrence (Edmonds *et al.* 1986). Patients with misshapen feet or who have had toes amputated will require bespoke shoes made for them by an orthotist.

Peripheral Vascular Disease

All patients with foot ulcers should have non-invasive vascular testing if no pulses are felt (Steed 1998). These tests may include ankle brachial pressure index (ABPI), although this result may be affected by calcification of the arteries (Reiber *et al.* 1998), or duplex ultrasound which gives both the anatomical and functional arteries. Digital subtraction arteriography can be thought of as the gold standard when it comes to vascular assessment of the tibial and foot vessels (Edmonds and Foster 1996).

The development of new techniques of re-vascularisation of the ischaemic foot has led to a reduction in the number of major amputations being performed on diabetics. Angioplasty should be the initial treatment of vascular disease where appropriate. Indications for angioplasty do not differ from the non-diabetic population, as studies have shown no differences in outcome between diabetics and non-diabetics (Davies *et al.* 1992).

Domain I – Management of Client Health/Illness Status

Immediate Management

The care assessment included a detailed history of Mr. C's foot ulcer. He explained that following surgery on his right foot last year he had been left with a fold in the skin. This had become increasingly painful over a period of eight weeks; he required increasing amounts of ibuprofen to relieve the pain. Eventually the fold in his skin split and started to ooze a clear fluid. At this point he sought help from his GP who prescribed oral antibiotics and a fungicidal cream, and arranged for the district nurse to dress the wound. It transpires that he had had several hospital admissions related to diabetic foot ulcers.

Examination of the right foot showed previous surgery and that his second toe had been amputated. There were also degenerative changes to this foot; a large wound covered the dorsum over the second and third metatarsal heads. Closer examination of the wound revealed a black necrotic area which was covering a piece of bone. The ability to probe bone is an indicator of osteomyelitis, and the probe indicated osteomyelitis was present (Grayson *et al.* 1990). The foot was hot to touch and there was a tract of cellulitis creeping up his limb. The foot was examined to see if pulses could be palpated; both the posterior tibial and dorsalis pedis pulses were palpable, which is an indicator that there was no significant ischaemia present in the foot. The vascular nurse practitioner contacted the vascular surgeons who arranged for a bed on the surgical unit at Newham General Hospital.

Once the foot had been assessed, the surgeons arranged for Mr C. to undergo amputation of his first and third toe. Mr C. was placed on intravenous antibiotics and the foot was closely observed. The fourth and fifth toe were not viable and the surgeons decided to perform a Syme's ankle disarticulation. This would allow Mr C. to have direct load transferring once the wound had healed (Pinzur 1999).

Modern dressings are designed to be left in place over a number of days. However, daily inspection is required for infected diabetic foot ulcers (Boulton *et al.* 1997; Vowden 1997). In fact Foster *et al.* (1994) has simplified the properties of a dressing that meets the need for the patient with diabetic foot ulcer, that is it does not take up too much space in the shoe; does not increase the risk of infection; absorbs exudate; and can be changed frequently. The Vascular Nurse Specialist liased with the ward nursing staff and surgeons to consider what dressing to use. It was decided to use a non-adherent dressing on the wound covered with saline soaked gauze and with wound pads; the dressing held in place using the a Kband bandage. This choice enabled the wound to be assessed on a daily basis and provided a non-adherent dressing for the wound bed (Jones 1998).

Ongoing Management

As a result of the Syme's procedure that Mr C. underwent, the podiatrist and orthotist felt the partial weight-bearing footwear was inappropriate. The Vascular Nurse Specialist and the surgeons arranged for Mr C. to be assessed at the local limb-fitting centre, who provided a patella tendon-bearing brace (Guse and Alvine 1997) which enabled Mr C. to commence early ambulation and be discharged home.

Prior to discharge, the Vascular Nurse Specialist liaised with the district nursing sister who would be looking after Mr C.'s foot wound and invited her into hospital to assess the wound and to observe the dressing technique. On discharge from hospital, the Vascular Nurse Specialist arranged for Mr C. to be assessed on a weekly basis at the joint podiatry and vascular nurses clinic.

Domain II – The Nurse–Client Relationship

Immediate Management

The Vascular Nurse Specialist visited Mr C. at home and arranged his admission into hospital. Following this admission, he offered support to Mr C. prior to his fore foot amputation. The VNS discussed why such a radical operation was necessary, that is to keep the wound open to allow it to heal by secondary intention, and also what the consequences to Mr C.'s mobility would be. Following the amputation the VNS re-emphasized to Mr C. why the foot wound had been left open and not *stitched-up*, explaining that the wound had been left open due to the sepsis in the foot and the wound would heal by secondary intention.

After a couple of days Mr C.'s mood became low and a long discussion with the VNS revealed that he blamed himself for the foot ulcer. Mr C. was worried about how long his recovery would take and frustrated by the fact he was unable to smoke as he was on bed rest. The VNS acknowledged that his hospital admission would be prolonged. It would be a lengthy period of time until he was able to mobilise on his limb, but without putting weight over his ulcer. Although Mr C. was aware that he should not weight bear on his ulcer, he was walking on it in order to smoke in the toilet. The dangers of his smoking were discussed at length with Mr C. He said that although he was aware of the dangers, smoking was his only pleasure and that he had no intention to stop smoking. Because of the damage Mr C. was causing to his ulcer, the VNS arranged for Mr C. to have a wheelchair so that he could go to the smoking room.

As previously stated, Mr C.'s sister died while he was in hospital. Mr C. was obviously very upset by this and wanted to attend the funeral. The VNS contacted the doctors who were looking after Mr C. so that he could attend the funeral and assisted with the booking of the transport to and from the funeral.

Ongoing Management

Mr C. was very unhappy with the patellar tendon-bearing brace. The VNS contacted the limb-fitting centre who explained that the brace was temporary, to prevent his body weight from bearing on the ulcer until it healed. Once the ulcer healed, Mr C. would receive a more cosmetically acceptable form of orthosis. The VNS explained this to Mr C. and, although unhappy with his current orthosis, he was pleased that this was not to be the final orthosis.

Most lesions in the foot occur following minor trauma. The initial pathway to major amputation is trauma resulting in cutaneous injury (Pecoraro *et al.* 1990). Therefore, it was vital that the VNS reinforced the importance to Mr C. of seeking help it he noticed a break in the skin, or the appearance of warmth, swelling, discharge or pain. Mr C. was given the Vascular Nurses contact number and encouraged to use it if he had concerns or questions.

As well as being given a contact number, Mr C. was seen on a weekly basis in the joint Podiatry and Vascular Nurse Specialist clinic for treatment of callus, ulcer debridement, assessment of how the wound was healing and to reinforce the foot care advice.

Domain III – The Teaching Coaching Function

Patient

Immediate Management

Mr C. required education about the continuing cause of his ulceration. Mantey *et al.* (1999) discussed the reasons why certain patients' ulcers recur. Patients with recurrent ulcers were shown to have a greater degree of peripheral neuropathy, poor diabetic control and to have a differing response to danger signs of the diabetic foot, compared to patients who did not have recurrent ulcers. This was Mr C.'s fourth admission in three years with diabetic foot ulcers, so it was important to assess what understanding Mr C. had with respect to foot ulcers. Mr C. was aware that he should check his feet on a daily basis, and that it was important to seek medical help as soon as injury occurred. Although Mr C. was able to recall this information, he had not taken any action until an ulcer had developed. He also admitted that he did not check his feet on a daily basis. Litchfield and Ramkissoon's (1996) findings were similar, with patients being able to recall advice given, but not always complying with that advice. A variety of techniques for patient education are available, but Edmonds *et al.* (1996) advocate the use of leaflets backed up by the spoken word.

Mr C. had already shown remorse about the condition of his foot, and the VNS felt that Mr C. was prepared to consider changing his behaviour. The education process took place over a number of weeks by reinforcing foot care advice, discussing the healing process of the ulcer and explaining the patella weight bearing prosthesis. Diabetic patients in Newham are given a leaflet produced by the British Diabetic Association which provides information about the care they should give to their feet. Mr C. was also seen by the Diabetic Nurse Specialist and the dietitian who gave him advice surrounding his diabetes and nutrition, respectively.

Ongoing management

Mr C. was evaluated weekly in the Joint Podiatry and Vascular clinic. On each visit the importance of following the advice to protect his feet was stressed. Edmonds (1987) has reported recurrence rates over a three-year follow-up period of 41 per cent and 35 per cent of neuropathic and neuroischaemic ulcers respectively. Once the ulcer was healed, Mr C. required regular assessment of his risk factors to prevent recurrence (Walsh 1995).

Health Care Professionals

Immediate management

The VNS visited Mr C. regularly when he was on the hospital ward, ensuring that diabetic foot protocol was followed. The district nurses provided one-to-one teaching when they visited Mr C. in hospital and on joint visits to him at home.

Ongoing management

In a review at Nottingham City Hospital Foot Clinic, it was estimated that substandard management of diabetic feet by healthcare professionals was twice as likely to contribute to the start or deterioration of lesions as carelessness on the part of the patient themselves (Jeffcoat and Marcfarlane 1995). In conjunction with the podiatrists, the VNS conduct teaching sessions for GP, community and hospital nurses, chiropodists and junior hospital doctors, which aim to raise the profile of diabetic foot disease and to encourage appropriate clinical management.

Domain IV – Professional Role

The Vascular Nurse Specialist arranged for Mr C. to use a wheelchair to provide access to the smoking room. Although smoking was detrimental to his foot, it had to be balanced with the fact that without the wheel chair Mr C. had been mobilising on his amputation in order to smoke, thereby, damaging his ulcer. This decision was made after Mr C. rejected assistance to stop smoking; he was quite adamant that this was his only pleasure. A review of smoking cessation techniques (Foulds 1996) showed that smokers who have no motivation to stop smoking are unlikely to benefit from health education and will continue to smoke. The VNS negotiated with Mr C. and he agreed that he would only use the wheelchair when he went for a cigarette and would not spend long periods in the chair, where the leg was not elevated and, therefore, at risk of developing oedema which could delay wound healing.

Domain V – Managing and Negotiating Health Care Delivery Systems

Immediate Management

The Vascular Nurse Specialist has been in post for approximately 14 months and in that time, with the Vascular Surgeons and podiatrists, has set up specialist clinics for the management of diabetic foot disease. It has taken time for GPs and district nurses to become aware of the clinic and the type of patient that should be referred to the service. Several teaching sessions have taken place with the local GPs and the VNS has visited various district nursing clinics to publicise the diabetic foot clinic. The number of patients being seen in each clinic is recorded and this information is used to negotiate further clinic time with health care managers.

The VNS works with patients in both a hospital and a community setting to provide continuity in their care. The vascular nurse specialist liaises closely with district nursing staff to ensure that the patients receive appropriate ulcer care. To this end, prior to Mr C.'s discharge, the district nursing sister was invited into the hospital to meet him and to observe Mr C.'s dressings.

Ongoing Management

The management of diabetic patients is ongoing and, because of the high recurrence rate, patients will always require follow up treatment for the rest of the lives. This places tremendous demands on the health service. However if the patient develops a diabetic foot ulcer the average annual cost of treatment is £3600; if the patient has to have an amputation the cost rises to £10 900 (McInnes *et al.* 1998). Together with the podiatrist, the VNS provides educational support to newly diagnosed diabetics and has increased in the number of ulcer clinics.

Domain VI – Monitoring and Ensuring the Quality of Health Care Practice

Immediate Management

The Vascular Nurse Specialist has developed protocols for hospital nursing staff for the management of diabetic foot ulcers. Teaching sessions have taken place for the nursing staff to enable them to follow these protocols.

Every patient referred to the VNS or seen in the diabetic foot clinic, has an individual record. These records include the standard patient details, where the patient was referred from, and if the patient is admitted into hospital, the length of stay for that patient. This information can be used for a number of activities, for example audit and business planning.

Ongoing Management

The VNS, along with the podiatrists, conducts audits among all patients that have been admitted with diabetic foot disease to see how many underwent amputation. The St Vincent Declaration (WHO, 1990) set a target for a reduction of amputation rates by 50 per cent through the progression of screening, education and development. These targets are being used as the benchmark for the diabetic foot team at Newham General Hospital.

References

Boulton, A., A. Knowles and N. Jackson (1997) 'Use of alginate and hydrocolloid in diabetic foot lesions', *Practical Diabetes International*, 14(5) p. 148

Caputo, G. (1994) 'Infection: Investigation and Management', in A. Boulton, H. Connor and P. Cavanagh (eds), *The Foot in Diabetes*, 2nd edn, Chichester, Wiley

Cotter, M. and N. Cameron (1997) 'The aetiopathogensis of diabetic neuropathy: metabolic theories', in A. Boulton (ed.), *Diabetic Neuropathy*, Carnforth, Marius Press

Cruse, P. and R. Foord (1973) 'A five year prospective study of 23,649 surgical wounds', *Arch Surgery*, 107(2) pp. 206–10

Davies, A., S. Cole, T. Magee, D. Scott, R. Bairon and M. Horrock (1992) 'The effect of diabetes mellitus on the outcome of angioplasty for lower limb ischaemia', *Diabetes Medicine*, 9(5) pp. 480–1

Edmonds, M. (1987) 'Experience in a multidisciplinary diabetic foot clinic', in H. Connor, A. Boulton and J. Ward (eds), The *Foot in Diabetes*, 1st edn, Chichester, Wiley

Edmonds, M., M. Blundell, M. Morris, E. Thomas, L. Cotton and P. Watkins (1986) 'Improved survival of the diabetic foot: the role of a specialised foot clinic', *Quarterly Journal of Medicine*, 60(232) pp. 763–71

Edmonds, M. and A. Foster (1998) 'Classification an Management Of Neuropathic and Neuroischaemic Ulcers', in A. Boulton, H. Connor and P. Cavanagh (eds), *The Foot in Diabetes*, 2nd edn, Chichester, Wiley

Edmonds, M. and A. Foster (1996) 'Diabetic Foot', in K. Shaw (ed.), *Diabetic Complications*, Chichester, Wiley

Edmonds, M., K. Van Acker and A. Foster (1996) 'Education and the Diabetic Foot', *Diabetic Medicine*, 13(1) pp. S61–S64

Foster, A., M. Greenhill and M. Edmonds (1994) 'Comparing two dressings in the treatment of diabetic foot ulcers', *Journal of Wound Care*, 3(5) pp. 224–8

Foulds, J. (1996) 'Strategies for smoking cessation', *British Medical Bulletin*, 52(1) pp. 157–73

Grayson, M., K. Balogh, E. Levin and A. Karchmer (1990) 'Probing to bone: a useful clinical sign for osteomyelitis in diabetic fetid feet', *Proceedings and Abstracts of the International Conference on Antimicrobial Agents and Chemotherapy*, Abstract No. 245, Washington DC, American Society of Microbiology

Guse, S. and F. Alvine (1997) 'Treatment of Diabetic Foot Ulcers and Charcot Neuroarthropathy: Using the Patellar Tendon-Bearing Brace', *Foot & Ankle International*, 18(10) pp. 675–8

Jeffcoat, W. and R. Marcfarlane (1995) *The Diabetic Foot*, London, Chapman and Hall Medical

Jones, V. (1998) 'Selecting a dressing for the diabetic foot: factors to consider', *The Diabetic Foot*, 1(2) pp. 48–52

Knowles, E. and N. Jackson (1997) 'Care of the diabetic foot', *Journal of Wound Care*, 6(5) pp. 227–30

Kumar, S., D. Fernando, A. Veves, E. Knowles, M. Young and A. Boulton (1991) 'Semmes–Weinstein 10g monofilament: a simple, effective and inexpensive screening device for identifying diabetic patients at risk of foot ulceration', *Diabetic Research and Clinical Practise*, 13(1–2) pp. 63–8

Kumar, S., H. Ashe, L. Parnell, D. Fernando, C. Tsigos, R. Young, J., Ward and A. Boulton (1994) 'The prevalence of foot ulceration and its correlates in type 2 diabetic patients: a population-based study', *Diabetic Medicine*, 11(5) pp. 480–4

Laing, P. (1998) 'The development and complications of diabetic foot ulcers', *American Journal of Surgery*, 176(2A) pp. 11s–19s

Litchfield, B. and S. Ramkissoon (1996) 'Foot-care education in patients with diabetes', *Professional Nurse*, 11(8) pp. 510–12

Mantey, I., A. Foster, S. Spencer and M. Edmonds (1999) 'Why do foot ulcers recur in diabetic patients?' *Diabetic Medicine*, 16(3) pp. 245–9

McInnes, A., J. Booth and I. Birch (1998) 'Multidisciplinary diabetic foot care teams: professional education', *The Diabetic Foot*, 1(3) pp. 109–15

Pavy, F. (1985) 'Introductory address to the discussion on the clinical aspects of glycosuria', *Lancet* ii, pp. 1085–7

Pecoraro, R., G. Reiber and E. Burgess (1990) 'Pathways to limb amputations: basis for prevention', *Diabetes Care*, 13(5) pp. 513–21

Pinzur, M. (1999) 'Restoration of walking ability with Syme's Ankle Disarticulation', *Clinical Orthopaedics and Related Research*, 361(1) pp. 71–5

Reiber, G., B. Lipsky and G. Gibbons (1998) 'The Burden of Diabetic Foot Ulcers', *American Journal of Surgery*, 176(2A) pp. 5s–10s

Renwick, P., K. Vowden, M. Wilkinson and P. Vowden (1998) 'The pathophysiology and treatment of the diabetic foot disease', *Journal of Wound Care*, 7(2) pp. 107–10

Rosenblum, R., F. Pomposelli, J. Giurini, G. Gibbions, D. Freeman, J. Chrzan, D. Campbell, G. Habershaw and F. LoGerfo (1994) 'Maximising foot salvage by a combined approach to foot ischaemia and neuropathic ulceration in patients with diabetes', *Diabetes Care*, 17(9) pp. 983–7

Steed, D. (1998) 'Foundations of Good Ulcer Care', *American Journal of Surgery*, 176(2A) pp. 20s–25s

Vowden, K. (1997) 'Diabetic foot complications', *Journal of Wound Care*, 6(1) pp. 4–8

Walsh, C. (1995) 'A healed ulcer: What Now?' *Diabetic Medicine*, 13(1) pp. S58–S60

WHO (World Health Organisation), Europe and International Diabetes Federation, Europe (1990), 'Diabetes care and research in Europe (St Vincent Declaration)', *Diabetic Medicine*, 7(4) p. 360

Index